WEAVING MINDFULNESS AND COMPASSION INTO YOGA TEACHING

in the same series

Theming Skills for Yoga Teachers
Tools to Inspire Creative and
Connected Classes
Tanja Mickwitz
ISBN 978 1 78775 687 8
eISBN 978 1 78775 688 5

Developing a Yoga Home Practice
An Exploration for Yoga
Teachers and Trainees
Alison Leighton with Joe Taft
ISBN 978 1 78775 704 2
eISBN 978 1 78775 705 9

Qigong in Yoga Teaching and Practice
Understanding Qi and the
Use of Meridian Energy
Joo Teoh
ISBN 978 1 78775 652 6
eISBN 978 1 78775 653 3

The Business of Yoga
A Guide to Starting, Growing and
Marketing Your Yoga Business
Katy Appleton and Natasha Moutran
ISBN 978 1 78775 642 7
eISBN 978 1 78775 643 4

**Supporting Yoga Students with
Common Injuries and Conditions**
A Handbook for Teachers and Trainees
Andrew McGonigle
ISBN 978 1 78775 469 0
eISBN 978 1 78775 470 6

Ayurveda in Yoga Teaching
Tarik Dervish
ISBN 978 1 78775 595 6
eISBN 978 1 78775 596 3

Series Editor Sian O'Neill

of related interest

Yoga Teaching Handbook
A Practical Guide for Yoga
Teachers and Trainees
Edited by Sian O'Neill
ISBN 978 1 84819 355 0
eISBN 978 0 85701 313 2

Yoga Student Handbook
Develop Your Knowledge of
Yoga Principles and Practice
Edited by Sian O'Neill
ISBN 978 0 85701 386 6
eISBN 978 0 85701 388 0

WEAVING MINDFULNESS AND COMPASSION INTO YOGA TEACHING

A Handbook for Teachers and Trainees

Anna Taylor

Foreword by Norman Blair
Illustrations by Masha Pimas

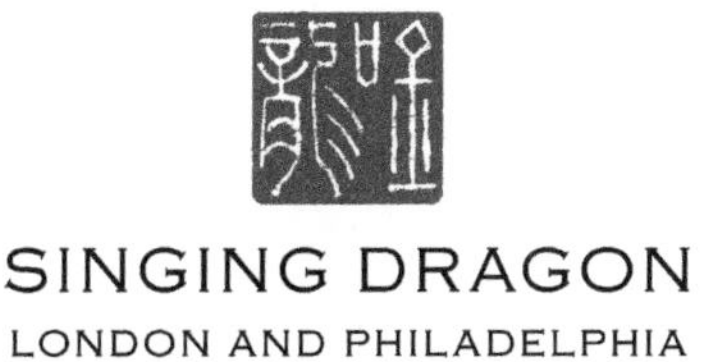

SINGING DRAGON
LONDON AND PHILADELPHIA

First published in Great Britain in 2025 by Singing Dragon,
an imprint of Jessica Kingsley Publishers
Part of John Murray Press

1

Copyright © Anna Taylor 2025

Illustrations by Masha Pimas

Front cover image source: Adrian Fisk. The cover image is for illustrative
purposes only, and any person featuring is a model.

A CIP catalogue record for this title is available from the
British Library and the Library of Congress

ISBN 978 1 78775 952 7
eISBN 978 1 78775 953 4

Printed and bound in Great Britain by CPI Group

Jessica Kingsley Publishers' policy is to use papers that are natural, renewable and recyclable
products and made from wood grown in sustainable forests. The logging and manufacturing
processes are expected to conform to the environmental regulations of the country of origin.

Singing Dragon
Carmelite House
50 Victoria Embankment
London EC4Y 0DZ

www.singingdragon.com

John Murray Press
Part of Hodder & Stoughton Limited
An Hachette UK Company

The authorised representative in the EEA is Hachette Ireland, 8 Castlecourt Centre,
Castleknock Road, Castleknock, Dublin 15, D15 YF6A, Ireland

CONTENTS

'This is important. What you are holding in your hands is crucial reading for all yoga teachers and all committed yoga practitioners…you will find jewels within these pages.'

– Norman Blair, author and yoga teacher

'As the foreword says, this book is important. Packed full of common-sense advice, as well as wide-ranging and accessible practical tools for teachers and students, it is an essential reminder that yoga is not about performance, but about giving ourselves space and time to really get to know ourselves, and to meet what we find with compassion, non-judgement and the willingness to change. An incredibly valuable resource for yoga teachers new and old.'

– Dr Graham Burns, yoga teacher and teacher trainer

'In the 21st century, the word *yoga* has become synonymous with the physical practice of yoga postures, relegating this time-tested spiritual technology to a form of calisthenics with Sanskrit names. Having jettisoned the essential values of yoga, modern practitioners are being short-changed of what could be a much deeper experience with rich rewards. Anna Taylor's *Weaving Mindfulness and Compassion into Yoga Teaching* reasserts that yoga's primary purpose is to reduce suffering and to awaken an awareness of ourselves and the world that is both clear and compassionate. What I love about this book is the warmth of the author's voice, which makes reading [it] feel like a warm balm for the soul. I highly recommend this accessible book, not only for yoga teachers, but for anyone interested in understanding yoga, themselves and what a yoga practice can be when it is re-connected to the heart of a living tradition.'

– Donna Farhi, author of Bringing Yoga to Life

'This wonderful book is filled with guidance and directions for not only practicing yoga mindfully but also taking this skill into daily living. It is an excellent resource for teachers for their own practice and sharing this wisdom with their students.'

– Bernie Clark, author and creator of YinYoga.com

'This book is a gift. Whether you've just qualified or you've decades of experience, you'll find insights on every page that will enrich and sustain your teaching practice. It's clear, inspiring and full of wisdom. I will be recommending it to every yoga teacher I know.'

– Naomi Annand, yoga teacher, teacher trainer and author of
Yoga: A Manual for Life *and* Yoga for Motherhood

'This book is born of experience. Centred around the transformation of self-critique and suffering into self-care and self-compassion, Anna Taylor draws equally on yoga and mindfulness practices and philosophy to knit together the methodologies and describe a body-heart-mind integrated approach to life. The text is alive with her authentic voice, sharing her experience and offering practice guidance to us readers on how to enliven physical practice with mindfulness, heart-felt curiosity and compassion. Anna illumines a path toward wholeness in language that is easy to understand and a pleasure to read. She leads us while standing right beside us.'

– Lisa Kaley-Isley, PhD, E-RYT 500, C-IAYT, clinical psychologist,
yoga therapist and yoga educator

FOREWORD

This is important. What you are holding in your hands is crucial reading for all yoga teachers and all committed yoga practitioners.

I have been teaching yoga since 2001, having begun practising in the early 1990s. In these 30 plus years, there have been considerable changes in this world, in my life, in yogaland (including its practice, teaching and culture). Some changes are positive – such as the diminishing of authoritarian guru structure and the growing awareness of our biological, psychological bodies. Some are negative – such as the increasing popularity of yoga as an aesthetic performance or, as Anna puts it, how 'social media can skew our perception so that we feel lost in a sea of competition rather than a valuable member of a community of teachers'.

This book, *Weaving Mindfulness and Compassion into Yoga Teaching*, is a clear sighted and thoughtful look at both the negative and positive changes. This is not a book that guarantees quick fixes. This is not a book of easy solutions. As Anna writes: 'Life can be complex and creating sustainable change is a gradual process.' Her aim is to help support yoga teachers and ensure that sustainability and integrity are more than words. She lays bare the undeniable facts that 'burn out is common' and 'the journey of self-exploration can be a bumpy one'.

Anna's approach is grounded in what could be described as open-source discussion. What she presents is an encouragement to ask questions, to consider what we are doing and to prioritize self-care. Over her years of practice and teaching, Anna has learned that mindfulness and compassion are more important than particular physical postures. If you are reading this book to find out how to make your hamstrings longer, then you will be disappointed. If you are reading this book to find out how you could be a better teacher, then you will find jewels within these pages.

Anna writes: 'As a yoga teacher, mindfulness and compassion have been central in enabling me to continue offering this work that I love.' These terms are skilfully explained in language that is accessible and bolstered by examples drawn from years of being on a yoga mat (and a meditation cushion). Anna has deeply studied these practices and she brings to their exploration here a great honesty. She is not afraid to acknowledge mistakes; she is not afraid to say that she did things differently in the past; she is not afraid to speak truths. 'If teaching is our sole revenue, there can be financial stresses with insecure and fluctuating incomes, no holiday or sick pay.'

Instead of being overwhelmed and undermined, instead of blind faith and dogmatic discipline, this is about creating spaces where yoga teachers can clearly discern what helps and what hinders, what inspires and what depletes, what nourishes and what exhausts. What can help us to 'guide students towards a state of presence', so that 'under these calmer conditions, we can learn and grow from our experiences rather than feeling stuck in or destabilized by them'. A space where yoga teachers are being empowered rather than being told what we to do. To quote Anna: 'It can feel a rare and precious gift to be offered space and permission to slow, still and quieten; to let our precious attention fold back inwards towards ourselves.'

Whether one is a new teacher or a highly experienced teacher, we can all learn from this skilfully woven book.

Norman Blair

ACKNOWLEDGEMENTS

This book has been made possible due to the support of so many.

I'm forever grateful to the numerous teachers that I've had the privilege to study with and be inspired by. There too many to name them all personally, but some that have been central to my journey and I would like to thank include Lisa Kaley-Isley (for your ongoing wisdom and support), Karen Atkinson (for championing the importance of compassion within mindfulness teaching and practice), Norman Blair (for your valued friendship, honesty and encouragement) and Monique Fryer (for being a constant beacon of light whatever weathers I'm navigating). Others who have been key in shaping both my practice and teaching include Tara Brach, Judith Hanson Lasater, Donna Farhi, Bo Forbes, Jack Kornfield, Kristin Neff, Naomi Annand and Ulla König.

When I think of the many different paths that life could have taken me on, I must also thank Janice Kate Fisher for planting the seed so many years ago that led to my taking a leap of faith and training to teach yoga.

I am deeply grateful to those who offered both time and reflective thoughts on draft versions of this book, particularly to Fritha Saunders and Maitripushpa Bois for helping to shape it in the editing stages, and to Graham Burns for providing support with Sanskrit terminology.

This book certainly would not have been possible without the love of my dear friends and family who encouraged and supported me through this process of writing (particularly when my own inner critic needed some external compassionate companions). There are too many to name individually, but you know who you are! I feel beyond lucky to move through the world with the loving safety net that you all provide.

I will always think fondly of Seal House in Selsey for the sea view that on so many occasions allowed my head to clear, my heart to open and words to flow during the process of writing.

Heart-felt thanks goes to all the wonderful students I've had the privilege of working with over the years. Your courage and commitment to stepping on the mat and offering yourself care and attention has moved me on so many occasions, as well as hearing your stories about how these practices have impacted your lives, both on and off the mat.

A special thanks also to Sian O'Neill for seeing something in my teaching that drew you to approach me about writing this book and to Singing Dragon for your support and patience in bringing it into fruition. Thanks also to Masha Pimas for bringing such warmth and heart to the illustrations.

INTRODUCTION

'Do you pay regular visits to yourself?'[1]

I love this question posed by the Sufi poet, Rumi.

For me, this is the essence of both yoga and mindfulness practice, offering precious time and space to meet ourselves; time to set aside the many roles and demands life places on us and open to what is right here and now in our inner and outer worlds.

An equally interesting question might be, 'When you do, what kind of visitor are you?' Are you a friendly one that is supportive and encouraging or one that is harsh and critical, forever pointing out your weaknesses? When preparing to pay a visit to ourselves, are we laying down a welcome mat or getting out a score card?

One of the achievements that I am most proud of in my life is learning to prioritize such visits. My practice, both on and off the mat, helps me to notice what type of visitor is present and how helpful they are (or aren't!) being.

The type of visitor I am to myself still spans a broad spectrum. It includes visitors who are fearful or eager to judge. But over the years, it has increasingly included other, more compassionate ones who are gentle and understanding, who offer care and warmth, who quietly accompany me during difficult times without telling me I am failing or feel they need to fix them immediately.

My practice offers space to step back and listen to each visitor. What is driving them? What are they needing? It allows me to notice how their company is impacting me, not just mentally but emotionally and physically; what patterns are playing out through my body, heart, mind. It helps me to see the causes and conditions that contribute to their arising, whether it be tiredness triggering one that is grumpy, or rest inviting a calm, considered one.

My hope is that this book will help both you and your students to also become more mindful and compassionate visitors when meeting yourselves through your yoga practice. The effects are then likely to ripple outwards, enabling us to become more compassionate companions toward others and the world that we live within.

Mindful, compassionate yoga for teachers and students

As a yoga teacher, mindfulness and compassion have been central in enabling me to continue offering this work that I love, reminding me to connect to what lights me up, to find steadiness when I wobble, to offer myself that which makes me feel resourced and supported while offering the same to others.

The paths of yoga and mindfulness share many common threads. Both offer space to explore our inner landscape as well as our relationship with the external world; both enable us to gain insights into our true nature, outside of the beliefs we might have about ourselves; both teach us to meet our varying experiences with greater calmness, clarity and equanimity.

The measures of success in both practices aren't found when we can stand on our heads nor focus on the breath undistracted for 30 minutes, but when we begin to move through life with greater presence of mind, ease of being and openness of heart, sensing the inherent interconnectivity between ourselves and the wider world that we live in. This book will explore the theory and offer practices to support you and your students.

In Section 1 we will explore what mindfulness and compassion are and how they interlink with yoga. Readers' prior knowledge of the subject will no doubt vary. For some, this may serve as a welcome reminder, for others a useful introduction.

In Section 2 we will explore how we, as practitioners who teach, can use mindfulness and compassion within our own lives to support both our wellbeing and the sustainability of our teaching. We will consider how they support us in practising self-care as well as caring for our students. It includes suggested practices and reflections to help you embed these tools within the varied aspects of teaching.

Section 3 explores ways of bringing mindfulness and compassion into the forefront of our yoga teaching in service of our students. Here, we will explore the whole of the teaching journey from intention setting to marketing, planning and directly teaching.

While many 200-hour teacher trainings offer detailed instruction on how to guide students into poses, fewer focus on how to guide students towards a state of presence. Here, we will explore this in depth, considering choices of sequencing, pacing, demonstrating and language use. This section includes a range of practices that can be incorporated within our teaching, both in movement and stillness. My suggestion is to explore and experiment with these in your own practice (noticing your own response – their impact, benefits and challenges) before sharing them with your students.

My journey

Over the years, as a practitioner and a teacher, I have absorbed many wonderful classes, teachings and trainings across a variety of traditions. I've discovered many gems that have sustained me and my teaching as I grow, age and change, but for me the most valuable elements of my practice have been mindfulness and compassion. But as is often the case, it's been quite a journey.

When I first stepped on a yoga mat in my mid-20s, yoga wasn't as mainstream as it is today. It was in an age before social media, so images of yoga weren't prevalent, and I'm now glad for that.

When I look back, I realize that the strong desire I felt to try yoga had no correlation to my understanding of what to expect when I did. What I do know is that I had huge hope. I hoped that it would help me to feel 'better'. I had neither the understanding nor the words to recognize in myself what was 'wrong' or what 'better' would look like, I just knew I had gotten a bit lost.

In my first class in a local school hall, I mistakenly walked into the 'advanced' class and was both bemused and confused by the sound of people chanting. I remember finding my way to the beginners' class and thinking it funny that the teacher was wearing skinny jeans (I now assume that she was having an 'off' day and had forgotten her teaching clothes). I remember not knowing what I was doing. I remember feeling into parts of my body that I'd not visited for years. I remember leaving feeling a bit 'better'.

As time continued, I flitted between different classes until I stumbled across a teacher whose gentle, quiet way held the big space and numerous students in a way that enabled me to both hide and feel seen in equal measure. As the years went by, I grew to understand that if I took myself to her class, however busy my mind, however self-critical the thoughts in my head, however weary my body felt, I would come out feeling 'better'.

I had no concept of how it worked, but over the years, I began to change. I became aware that my body held things my mind didn't always process: tensions, emotions, wisdom. I learnt that my mind wasn't always telling the truth and discovered a new, deeper sense of wisdom than the mental chatter of my everyday life. I found there was another calmer, clearer version of myself that often felt hidden from view but would surface towards the end of class and I would carry her with me out into the world with a greater sense of ease and balance.

What I can see now, many years later, is how disconnected I had become from my body. I lived my life in my busy mind and tried to solve all my perceived problems and inadequacies with my head, which often left me feeling more tangled, jangled, exhausted and defeated. Pausing, quietening and listening inward were unfamiliar territory to me but somehow the calm, grounded, compassionate space held by this teacher made it a safe space within which to explore it.

Weekly classes soon expanded into a daily personal practice. Something was shifting and changing. It was a slow and often subtle process but there was a magic in this practice – it felt like a medicine that needed to be taken in regular doses.

I never dreamed of becoming a yoga teacher. I assumed that this was a role set aside for people far more sorted than myself. I remember commenting to my teacher about how rewarding teaching must be and her suggesting that I train to do so. I initially met her words with incredulous resistance — but something in them landed, like a seed that had hit fertile soil but just needed the right time and conditions to take root.

For most of my life, I had reached into my rational, thinking mind to make all major decisions, but as my mental chatter increasingly quietened, I learnt to better detect, decipher and trust in this quieter, wiser, deeper wisdom. When life's conditions changed, this gentle but persistent inner voice (that resided as much in my body as my mind) brought that seed to life and I stepped into my first yoga teacher training.

As teachers, we are first and foremost students and practitioners. Many of us invest vast amounts of time and energy (not to mention money) in our continued learning. I spent my first few years of teaching reaching into a range of trainings, partly led by a desire to deepen my learning, partly led by my insecurities that I was not 'good enough'. I explored and experimented with different styles and trainings, until it became increasingly clear it was the therapeutic aspect of yoga that my heart was drawn to, and I began my training as a yoga therapist.

It was during this time that meditation became a deeper part of my practice. My introduction to meditation many years earlier had offered unpromising beginnings. In a beautiful Buddhist retreat centre in Scotland, my friend banished me from sitting next to her: my head nodding was distracting as I dozed off during the 7 am sittings. But years later, here on the yoga mat, the importance of cultivating a compassionate presence was deepening as was my need to create space for quietness and stillness.

I remember devouring Tara Brach's book *Radical Acceptance*,[2] which offered a path for meeting myself with greater awareness and compassion. It felt such a relief to read that my busy, self-critical mind wasn't abnormal but that there were practices that could allow me to meet myself differently. Their power, their capacity to change how I connected to and cared for myself, was palpable as I wove them into my practice. It became increasingly clear how essential these qualities were in creating positive therapeutic relationships with my clients; how much healing occurs when we feel truly seen, heard and compassionately held; how transformative simple practices can feel when undertaken with a tender, caring attention.

Although our journeys to teaching are all unique, many of us share a similar path. We experience the benefits of practice in our own lives and feel a pull to share them with others. The more we learn about these powerful practices, the more we realize how little we know. It is a journey that can be both inspiring and daunting; it brings with it responsibilities and insecurities as well as being a humbling, heart-warming privilege to hold space for others' journeys.

My own journey is forever ongoing. I continue to reach into these practices daily because I need them. I am human, I make mistakes, life can be wobbly and confusing. Being a yoga teacher doesn't make us enlightened nor superhuman, but rather people on a path, sharing what we are learning.

What this book is and what it is not

As teachers, we come from a broad range of yoga lineages and we bring with us our unique life experiences, voices and styles of teaching; this is to be celebrated. What is important is that we teach that which resonates with us, from a place of authenticity. My hope is that this book offers you space for exploration and reflection, enabling you to teach from a place that inspires and nourishes you. This book does not suggest a definitive way that yoga should be taught but rather it offers suggestions and space for reflection.

It is important to stress that this book is *not* a guide for teaching mindfulness and compassion courses to groups or individuals. Should this be your focus, I would strongly recommend undertaking a training with a provider who is approved and registered with an appropriate professional body (e.g., British Association for Mindfulness-based Approaches (BAMBA) in the UK and the European Associations for Mindfulness (EAMBA) within Europe). The focus here is to support you as yoga teachers in having a deeper understanding of what mindfulness and compassion are and how you can apply this within the context of yoga teaching.

My suggestion is to read the book sequentially, enabling you to explore, embed and embody mindfulness and compassion into your own life and practice before sharing them with your students. That said, Section 3 includes a range of tools and considerations when teaching others that you may like to explore within your own practice.

The teachings of yoga, mindfulness and compassion are vast and forever evolving. I am not an academic scholar of either Buddhist or yoga traditions but rather a fellow teacher who has found great value in these teachings and a desire to share how I use them. My hope is that this book will encourage you to weave these gem-like threads of mindfulness and compassion into your life and teaching to enhance both your and your students' experiences.

A note on Sanskrit terminology

I am grateful to Graham Burns for offering the following notes on Sanskrit terminology:

Because the Sanskrit alphabet has many more letters than our 'western' alphabets, a number of conventions have been devised to represent Sanskrit words consistently into western script. In this book, we have adopted the International Alphabet of Sanskrit Transliteration (IAST) system, which uses a range of dots, dashes and other symbols (collectively known as 'diacritics') above and below certain letters.

For readers wishing to learn accurate pronunciation of Sanskrit words, the pronunciation guide in the table below may be helpful. All other letters in Sanskrit words should be pronounced broadly as in English.

Letter/diphthong	Pronunciation
a	as in Southern English cup (*not* cap)
ā	as in palm
e	as in bale (*not* bell)
i	as in bit
ī	as in beak
o	as in cope (*not* cop)
u	as in butt
ū	as in tool
ai	as in aisle (*not* hail)
au	as in cow
c	as in chat (*not* cat)

cont.

Letter/diphthong	Pronunciation
ḥ	a soft echo of the preceding vowel
j	as in joke (*not* yolk)
jñ	as in igneous (though with a slightly softer g sound)
kṣ	as in action
ṃ	as in the French word bon (i.e., nasal)
ṅ	roughly as in king, without the 'g' (i.e., nasal)
ñ	as the 'ny' sound in onion when before a vowel; as in angel when before a consonant
ṇ	as in pan, but with the tongue turned back lightly to the roof of the mouth
ph	as in cuphook (*not* flower)
ṛ	as r with a short i after it (e.g., as in rip)
ṣ	as in push, but with the tongue turned back lightly to the roof of the mouth
ś	as in shout
ṭ	as in tea, but with the tongue turned back lightly to the roof of the mouth
th	as in pothook (*not* theatre)
ṭh	as in pothook, but with the tongue turned back lightly to the roof of the mouth
v	half way between the English v and w sounds: can be sounded as either English letter

WHY MINDFULNESS AND COMPASSION

'The success of Yoga does not lie in the ability to perform postures but in how it positively changes the way we live our life and our relationships.'

TKV Desikachar[1]

Overview

Mindful, compassionate awareness lies at the heart of our yoga practice. It is not something to layer on, but rather an integral thread woven within. Inherent within our practice is opening to the present moment, gently exploring, inquiring and reflecting on the nature of our experience (*svādhyāya* in Sanskrit), deepening our understanding of ourselves, our true nature and our place in the wider world.

While modern images of yoga may suggest that the fruits of our practice are found in physical forms, in *Sūtra* 1.2 of the *Yoga Sūtras* (one of the foundational texts on yoga) Patañjali defines yoga as *yogaścittavṛt-tinirodhaḥ*, often translated as 'yoga is the stilling or controlling of the fluctuations of the mind'. Yoga, therefore, is a state of mind, one that is steady, stable, free from distractions and distortions, the mind 'stuff' that so often skews our perception and contributes to our suffering. We might think of yoga then as both a state of being and a path guiding us towards it.

For many of us, the physical poses (*āsana*) within our practice offer a useful vehicle for cultivating presence. Feeling our feet against the ground and the breath flowing through us can feel a welcome relief when often lost in thought, steering our busy minds into the here and now. While our bodies play a vital role in meeting ourselves on the mat, the poses serve a purpose rather than being the goal of our practice. Equally as important as 'training' our bodies (to be steady and spacious) is training our hearts and minds (to be open, compassionate, stable and clear seeing). In the words of Ranju Roy and David Charlton, 'If there is no change in our mental state when we practice, there has been no yoga, no matter how beautiful or elaborate our postures'.[2]

While yoga is sometimes labelled as a practice of 'love and light' what draws most of us to the mat is a desire to feel 'better'. 'Suffering' (*duḥkha*) can seem a big word, one reserved for life's catastrophic events, but when viewed as a sense of discontent or dissatisfaction, we can see how it plays out in various shapes and forms within our lives. Sometimes, it appears as a subtle grumbling found in an achy shoulder or a tired and grumpy mind, at other times life events shake us to our core and it dominates our lives. However we phrase it, whether small or big, subtle or strong, it is often a desire to reduce suffering that draws us towards our yoga practice.

Both the paths of Buddhism (from which the explicit emphasis on mindfulness is considered to originate) and yoga stem from the understanding that much of our suffering arises from a lack of clear seeing or misapprehension (*avidyā*). Our brains are more concerned with our survival than our happiness, and so steer how we perceive and respond to the world with that focus. While helpful in keeping us alive, this isn't always conducive to feelings of peace and ease (nor the insights and wisdom that can arise in calmer conditions). Both traditions shine a light on habits of mind that skew our perception while offering paths to living with greater clarity and peace.

Chapter 1

WHAT IS MINDFULNESS?

The English term 'mindfulness' was coined by Jon Kabat-Zinn, often thought of as the founder of modern mindfulness. As a long-term practitioner of both yoga and Buddhist meditation and a Professor at the University of Massachusetts Medical School, he recognized the benefits these mind/body practices could have for his patients suffering with chronic health conditions, their potential to improve wellbeing and ease stress and suffering.

It was while on retreat with the Buddhist monk Thich Nhat Hanh that the inspiration came to him to devise a programme combining awareness-based meditation and yoga practices that would be accessible to a more secular audience. The eight-week Mindfulness Based Stress Reduction (MBSR) programme was born in 1979 and, due to scientific evidence gathered on the benefits that participants gained, secular mindful meditation began to spread more widely in the West.

While 'mindfulness' may be a modern term, it has been practised for thousands of years and lies at the heart of many spiritual traditions. It is a quality of presence, one in which we open to our present moment experience with an open, caring, non-judgemental awareness. We can direct it outwardly – opening our senses to sights, sounds, smells, tastes, textures as we interact with others and the world around us. We can direct it inwardly – tuning into the sensations in our bodies, the thoughts and feelings moving through our minds and hearts.

There is an image I love that's often used to illustrate the contrast between moving through the world in a way that is mindful or, as we often do, with our minds full. It shows a person and a dog walking through a park. Thought bubbles reflect the nature of their minds: the dog's fully present to the moment before them, aware of the trees, sky and sun that it is walking towards; the person's, however, is crammed full of thoughts – the work to be done, the calls to be made, the bills to be paid – oblivious to the beauty before them.

Many of us can relate to this image, asking ourselves: 'How often does our mind feel like the dog's, being truly present to the life that is before us? How often does it feel like the person's, filled with busy thoughts?' We might recognize the nature of our own thought bubbles as we arrive to teach, juggling the demands of life as we step on the mat ourselves. We might appreciate the nature of many students' minds as they arrive in our class. Life happens. We are human. It is a complicated combination.

So often we live our lives in a mode of 'doing', forever trying to fix, change or achieve something. Even when we press pause from physical activity our minds are often intent on leaping to action through thinking, daydreaming, planning, etc. Mindfulness steers us towards a mode of 'being' with our experience, opening to, allowing, exploring what is right here before us (and within us) without trying to immediately shape it.

Shifting into 'being' mode can sometimes feel calming. I often sense my body soften and my breath deepen as I let go of pushing up against how things are or battling for things to be a certain way. However, it's important to recognize that mindfulness isn't a relaxation technique; we are not trying to create any particular state, rather we are learning to be more present and less reactive to what we are experiencing.

While the word '*mind*fulness' can suggest a solely cognitive, mental process, this is not the case. In many traditions, a distinction isn't made between mind and heart (nor mind and body). The Sanskrit word '*citta*' refers to both mental and emotional states, so we might think of it as heart/mind. In this context, mindfulness could more accurately be thought of as a *heartful* awareness; one that connects us as deeply to our somatic, embodied and emotional experience as much as our mental processes.

While mindfulness is a form of meditation, its practice isn't limited to the mat or meditation cushion. In the Buddha's teachings, he was clear that it could be practised in any moment of our lives, whether sitting, lying down, standing or moving. After all, our goal isn't to get better at touching our toes or noticing our breath, but to navigate our everyday lives with greater skill and awareness.

Although mindfulness is considered a secular practice, I would argue that it is inherently a spiritual one. In seeing the nature of life more clearly, we become aware of our deep interconnectedness. We sense this internally, how our body, mind, heart and spirit are intrinsically interlinked; a pleasant thought can bring a feeling of joy which might soften the body and bring a lightness of spirit. We become aware of how intrinsically connected we are to each other and the wider world we live in. This can offer us a sense of belonging to something bigger than our small selves, whether that be our community, nature, the universe or our faith if we follow a religious path. It can help us recognize that our personal peace isn't obtained in isolation but rather through cultivating caring connections or loving kindness (*metta*) towards all beings. In doing so, mindfulness steers us in the direction of compassionate action and an ethical way of living.

Mindfulness, therefore, is much more than simply paying attention; after all, a bank robber is a master of being alert and attentive, but they're not an example of mindfulness in action.

Mindful awareness within our yoga practice

Mindfulness awareness is woven throughout our yoga practice. If we consider the 8 Limbs outlined by Patañjali in the *Yoga Sūtras,* we can see how they guide us to become more aware of both our inner and outer worlds as well as offering ways of navigating them with greater peace, clarity and caring connection.

The 8 Limbs offer a systematic path guiding us towards deeper states of meditative absorption, moving from that which is more tangible towards that which is more subtle. As with many texts, translations, spellings and definitions vary, and here I've drawn on translations offered by Roy and Charlton,[1] which resonate with me. In simplistic terms we might see these as:

- *YAMAS*: Bringing awareness to our relationships (both with ourselves and others), lessening tendencies that create discord and harm and so practicing: *ahiṃsā*, often translated as non-violence, is our intention that our actions (in thought, speech and deeds) are not harmful; *satya*, often translated as truthfulness, asks us to express ourselves authentically and truthfully; *asteya*, often translated as non-stealing, might be seen as not taking that which isn't ours to have (including inappropriately taking another's time or attention); *brahmacarya*, often translated as moderation (and in monastic settings, sometimes relates to conserving vital energy through celibacy), could be seen as staying focused on what matters, rather than our vital energy being dissipated through unhelpful desires, excess and over stimulation; and *aparigraha*, often translated as non-grasping, might be seen as not grasping for things to be a certain way, but rather being open to how things are.

- *NIYAMAS*: Bringing awareness to how we relate and tend to ourselves and our lives and cultivating habits that are conducive with greater clarity and peace and so practicing: *śauca*, often translated as cleanliness, but could be seen as self-care; *saṃtoṣa*, often translated as contentment, but could be seen as being at ease within ourselves; *tapas*, often translated as discipline, reflects the consistent effort required to change habitual patterns through our practice; *svādhyāya*, often translated as self-study, reflects our capacity to pay attention, inquire and reflect on the nature of our experience; and *īśvarapraṇidhāna*, often translated as devotion or surrendering to a higher power. Roy and Charlton's definition really resonates with me that this reflects 'a trust in the process of Life, [and] requires that we consider our relationship to forces beyond our control, and our place within the greater world order'.[2]

- *ĀSANA*: Bringing awareness to the body, cultivating qualities of steadiness (*sthira*), spaciousness and ease (*sukha*), supporting greater comfort and accessibility to maintain a steady, spacious posture and quality of awareness during prolonged periods of stillness and meditation.

- *PRĀṆĀYĀMA*: Bringing awareness to the more subtle energetic body, noticing and shaping the flow of *prāṇa* (vital life force) via the breath, in order to focus and steady the mind, creating the conditions for meditation.

- *PRATYĀHĀRA*: Roy and Charlton offer that '*pratyāhāra* is not a practice, but rather a state arising from our meditative focus. Prāṇāyāma is the primary means to cultivate this interiorised state'.[3] As we begin to be able to focus and refine our attention towards our inner experience, we become less distracted by our senses and external conditions.

- *DHĀRAṆĀ*: Here, we move closer towards a state of meditation by developing a focused concentration on an object of awareness (e.g., sounds, the body, the breath). While at this stage, our quality of presence will waver, we repeatedly guide our attention back to our object of focus, to stabilize it.

- *DHYĀNA*: Here, in a state of meditation, our connection to our object of focus remains steady, deepening our capacity to see the object clearly and gain insights into its true nature.

- *SAMĀDHI*: Here, in a state of meditative absorption, we experience a sense of oneness with the object of focus. Here, the mind is clear and stable, able to discern the object's true nature with clarity. We might consider this to be a state of mindful awareness.

These principles can be woven within a teaching setting, drawing students towards cultivating a mindful presence through their practice, moving from that which is more tangible to that which is more subtle.

While the *yamas* and *niyamas* offer guidance on how to meet ourselves and others in life, they can equally be applied to the mat and meditation cushion, ensuring that our practice offers space for exploration and inquiry (over performance and perfectionism), for caring and nourishing (over pushing and punishing), for connecting to our truth and learning to express it, for cultivating a disciplined effort, for opening to ourselves as we are and appreciating what we have rather than forever grasping for more, learning to cultivate positive habits while also accepting aspects that are beyond our control.

As we incorporate qualities of mindfulness within our *āsana* practice, it becomes mindfulness in motion (as well as stillness). For many, movement offers a more accessible starting point for presence, connecting to the body in a way that is closer to our everyday lived experience, therefore, is more familiar.

Āsana practice often offers more concrete sensations to direct our attention to (e.g., tuning into more perceptible sensations of stretch, engagement, contraction, expansion, pressure, release).

Without adequate preparation, being still can be challenging, our minds easily distracted by discomfort in the body and a mind intent on thinking. Particularly when our lives are busy, mindful movement can help to dissipate stress hormones rather than them coursing through us making us feel agitated, fidgety and fizzy in stillness.

In holding poses for several breaths (rather than 5–20 minutes, unless practising more still forms of yin and restorative yoga), we build our capacity for stillness gradually, from shorter to more prolonged periods.

That said, our *āsana* practice serves the purpose of guiding us more comfortably *towards* stillness rather than replacing it. In an age where so much value is placed on activity and productivity, it is easy for our yoga practice to follow suit, with *āsana* dominating our teaching and practice and only limited periods offered to the stillness of *prāṇāyāma, Śavāsana* and still forms of meditation.

For many students, their practice is the only time in which they have space to pause and quieten without zoning out or trying to fill it. Our practice guides us towards becoming increasingly comfortable and focused within prolonged periods of stillness. As the chatter in our minds quietens, valuable insights can arise within the quiet space between activities; therefore, it can be helpful to become more comfortable in offering this to both ourselves and our students.

Practising presence

'Being present' can sound simple but it is often surprisingly challenging, our brain eager to steer our mind in different directions. Even when we *intend* to pay attention, we find our mind has other ideas, delving into the past and leaping into the future, problem solving and planning.

Minds are made to both wonder and wander and, without training, their default mode is to dart here and there. I remember one of my first teachers explaining how our mind is like a drunken monkey that has been bitten by a scorpion. In today's world, it also has a smart phone in its hand, hooked on stimulation.

Unless we consciously create time to practise presence, our lives are easily lived with an absence of it. Much of the time, we are living our lives on 'auto-pilot', going through our daily activities but lost in thought. We've probably all had a journey where we have found our way home but have no recollection of the journey. While helpful at times to avoid sensory overload, being in this mode *all* the time means we miss much of the depth and detail of our lives.

Even when we *do* pay attention, our perception (and subsequent responses) is often skewed by unconscious forces rather than the reality before us. Rather than viewing the world before us as it is, the brain saves time and energy by filling in gaps, viewing it through the filter of our past experience, our beliefs, social norms and conditioning. Hence, five people can witness the same event but have wildly different perceptions and recollections of it. Similarly, the same conditions can seem difficult when we are tired and more manageable when we are happy.

Deepening our capacity for mindful presence (a mind that is stable, focused and clear seeing), therefore, requires a commitment to persistent practice. It is not a quick fix. Patañjali outlines that achieving this state of yoga requires regular practice (*abhyāsa*). It also requires kindness and patience, particularly when what we meet is different to how we would wish it to be.

The Buddhist term for mindfulness, '*sati*' in Pāli (the language of the Buddhist Pāli Canon), can be translated as 'to remember'. I find this helpful to acknowledge that mindfulness is not a permanent state that we perfect, but rather something that we remember to return to. We needn't berate ourselves when our mind wanders from presence; it is natural that does (and often!), but we can notice when it has and commit to regularly unhooking ourselves from our habitual thinking and tuning into what we are directly experiencing.

With mindfulness at the heart of our yoga practice, it becomes less something we are 'doing' and more time and space for 'being', an opportunity to press pause from our tasks, roles and duties and come home to ourselves, enabling us to see more clearly and respond more wisely to our internal and external conditions.

These regular pockets of 'non-doing' slowly seep into our everyday living, enabling us to feel more focused, clear-minded and easeful within the 'doing' parts of our day. In the words of Thich Nhat Hanh: 'Doing nothing brings about quality of being, which is very important. So doing nothing is actually doing something.'[4] Something we can remind ourselves of if the idea of doing nothing makes us feel indulgent or guilty!

The power of pausing

A key aspect of mindfulness is cultivating our capacity to pause. The power of pausing is captured beautifully in the words of the psychiatrist (and Holocaust survivor) Viktor Frankl: 'Between stimulus and response there is a space. In that space is our power to choose our response. In our response lies our growth and our freedom.'[5]

Particularly when we feel triggered or caught in strong emotions, our minds can get caught in fear-based modes of thinking, steering us to defend, attack, retreat or freeze. Our capacity to pause enables us to step out of auto-pilot and our habitual conditioning. It creates space between what is happening and our response to it. In this space, we can see it more clearly, meet it more calmly and hold it more kindly. Under these steadier, more compassionate conditions, our nervous system calms and we can respond from a place of wise discernment rather than habitual reactivity.

I have felt this in myself so many times in my own life. Whether for a few breaths, moments, minutes or an extended period, deepening my capacity to pause helps me meet and respond to my life very differently. As space opens and I take a moment to feel my feet on the ground and the breath flowing though me, I can soothe myself enough to meet and respond to the situation more calmly.

Cultivating a witness presence

Seeing clearly often requires us to step back a little, creating sufficient distance to become more of a witness to our experience. While the term 'non-attachment' (*vairāgya*) may seem somewhat cold or disinterested, implying a lack of connection, this isn't the intention.

Instead, we can think of it as 'untangling from', creating the conditions where we feel less overly identified with our experience. This enables us to hold it in a more spacious awareness, exploring it from different perspectives rather than being stuck in one outlook. We can hold our experience with sufficient spaciousness that we needn't be immediately reactive towards it. This can offer the space to see more clearly and respond with wisdom and discernment.

Particularly if what we are observing is ourselves (e.g., a tight shoulder or our anger), this can help us to meet our experience more objectively, rather than feeling so defined by it or needing to defend it.

We often consider our sense of self as consisting of 'I', 'me', 'mine', e.g., '*I* am thinking X', '*my* body is feeling hot', 'you did that to *me*'. The teachings of both the Buddha and Patañjali highlight how this over-identification with 'I', 'me' and 'mine' can create much of our suffering. Within the *Yoga Sūtras* this egocentric way of perceiving ourselves (*asmitā*) forms one of the *kleśas*, the mental habits that cloud our clear perception (the overriding one being that of *avidyā*, our lack of clear seeing) and add to our suffering.

Having a healthy sense of self or ego isn't bad, it can lead to healthy boundaries and self-care. Non-attachment is not about dissolving our sense of self, but being less identified with it and understanding the true nature of it. With mindful attention, we begin to sense that our 'self' as we often think of it (body, heart, mind) is not a fixed, solid state, but rather one of shift and change. Rather than feeling inflated by 'our' gains and devastated by 'our' losses, we sense the impermanent nature of experiences – the breath comes and goes, the body grows and decays, thoughts and feelings arise and pass. We sense that while these layers of body, heart, mind form part of our experience and are worthy of our care and attention, they are not the defining element of us.

As we step back and observe from this 'witness' perspective, we sense that we are more than this body, heart and mind (that are forever in a state of flux and change). We sense that our true nature is the steady, spacious awareness that *observes* our experience. We see this reflected in the *Yoga Sūtras* as Patañjali outlines our true Self is *puruṣa*, the unchanging witnesses consciousness that observes our experience but we suffer when we confuse our identity with *prakṛti*, the 'objects' of our awareness (e.g., the body, the mind and other elements of experience) that are transient and subject to change.

While this can seem somehow lofty and abstract, we might sense how this plays out in our practice, how different it feels to pay attention to sensations moving *through the* body, thoughts moving *through the* mind and emotions moving *through the* heart, opening to them without feeling so defined by them. A student of mine once put this so beautifully after a practice. She said that she became aware of two aspects of herself: one that was hurting and another that felt like a kind witness observing and holding her experience.

Pathways to presence

Given the wayward nature of our minds, many meditative traditions recognize the value of having 'anchors' to rest our attention on, offering a clear pathway back to presence when our attention veers from it. Both in movement and stillness, our yoga practices offers a variety of pathways to presence, including:

Senses

In opening to our environment, we 'come to our senses', tuning into the sights, sounds (even smells, tastes or textures) presented by an object or our environment. This is sometimes referred to as developing our capacity for 'exteroception'.

Particularly if tuning inwards feels overwhelming, resting our attention on something external, like a soundscape, can be helpful, being less emotionally charged than our inner experience.

Within our practice, we also tune into our relationship *with* our environment – our contact points with the ground and space surrounding us – strengthening our sense of where we are in space, cultivating our capacity for 'proprioception'.

The body

As we draw our attention away from the external world towards our internal experience we develop our capacity for 'interoception'.

In cultures that place higher value on cognitive function over embodied awareness, many of us spend our lives 'lost in thought', somewhat estranged from our bodies. As we practise with mindful awareness, we learn to reconnect with these living, breathing homes that we move through life in.

Rather than thinking about or analysing our body, we tune into our direct, sensory experience of it. While our thoughts tend to carry us back to the past and into the future, our physical sensations always reside in the present moment. We *feel* our heart beating and breath flowing, we experience qualities of opening, softening, engaging and contracting, sensations of cold, heat, tingling, and even noticing places where we experience numbness or lack of sensation.

Our practice offers us insights into our relationship with our bodies. Is our relationship a friendly one? Are we connecting to, listening to, loving and nourishing these bodies? Or are we ignoring, berating or even battling with them? Are there places calling for our attention or places we zone out from, patterns of holding so habitual we no longer notice them? Our answer will likely vary day-to-day, through ups and downs, illness and health.

When practised mindfully, our yoga practice is, therefore, about so much more than 'using' or 'doing' poses with our bodies, it is about reconnecting to them, learning to embody them, listen to them, tend to them and, dare we consider it, even enjoy, befriend and feel grateful for them. At times we may need or seek strong sensations to be able to 'feel' anything, but over time our capacity to tune into subtlety deepens.

While reconnecting to our bodies can feel like coming home for some, for others the body may not feel a safe refuge to occupy. Our bodies hold the patterns of our lived experience and, as the saying goes, 'our issues are in our tissues'. If we have experiences of trauma, reconnecting with the body often needs to be undertaken slowly, skilfully and sensitively. Exploring trauma-sensitive approaches to both yoga and mindfulness may be helpful if this is the experience of either yourself or your clients.

As well as moving mindfully in our *āsana* practice, The Body Scan and the Compassionate Body Scan are lovely practices that use the body as the main anchor for our awareness (see Section 3).

The breath

The breath is another common anchor in many meditative traditions. While the breath is always with us, it often lies beneath our conscious awareness. Through our practice, we can bring it to the foreground, tuning into the felt sense of it. We become attuned to its rhythms, speed, texture and depth, how it changes according to our internal and external conditions, through movement and stillness. We notice sensations of expansion and contraction, shifts in temperature as it enters and leaves the body, noticing where it flows with ease and places where it is limited.

Within our yoga practice, we often consciously shape our breath, slowing, smoothing and lengthening it. Within our *prāṇāyāma* practice, we intentionally manipulate the breath for specific benefits (e.g., to enliven, calm or balance our nervous system). Bringing a mindful attention to our *prāṇāyāma* practice helps us to be attentive to its impact, ensuring that we practice skilfully, tailoring it to our individual needs.

Within our mindfulness practice, however, we simply observe the natural breath as we find it rather than trying to shape it. In my own experience, the act of noticing my breath often changes it a little, slowing and smoothing it slightly, but this comes naturally rather than by forcing it. It is like we are watching ourselves being breathed rather than 'doing' the breathing.

Allowing moments to simply observe the breath within our yoga practice offers us valuable insights into habitual breathing patterns and their impact on body and mind. When we are at ease, our breath is often slower, smoother, with movement sensed in the abdomen. When we are stressed or overexerting, it can become faster, shorter and restricted to the chest cavity. Our breath, therefore, becomes like a barometer, offering an indication of our internal weather system both on and off the mat.

Practices that offer the breath as an anchor include Mindfulness of Breathing and Compassionate Breathing (see Section 3).

Thoughts and emotions

While thoughts can sometimes be perceived as an intrusive visitor, they aren't an enemy of our practice. We're not seeking to clear our mind of thoughts, but rather to see clearly when we are 'lost' in them and become more skilful in working with them (rather than always believing them or immediately acting on them).

At times, we might intentionally place qualities of heart/mind in the foreground of our attention, developing our capacity to both notice and name them, sensing patterns within them, the causes and impact of them.

We might notice familiar patterns, such as 'planning', 'ruminating' or 'berating', sensing whether they are helpful or harmful. As we wobble in a balancing pose, do we judge ourselves? As we rest in *Śavāsana*, does a feeling of ease or relief arise? As we rest over a bolster, do feelings of guilt come up? Our practice offers space to notice our thoughts, question their validity and cultivate new, more supportive qualities of heart/mind where these are helpful. I remember a client announcing her surprise and delight when a new, more compassionate voice arose in her practice, instead of the one that forever told her, 'You're rubbish'.

As we step back from our thoughts, learning to hold them more spaciously, we sense that our thoughts aren't necessarily facts, but rather mental events, that much like physical sensations they arise and pass when we stop feeding them through layering on additional narratives and judgements. Similarly, when strong emotions arise, we learn to hold them tenderly, reducing the tendency to feel so overwhelmed or defined by them.

After all, liberation comes not from freeing ourselves from our thoughts and feelings, but rather in freeing ourselves from believing or being defined by them. In the words of Jack Kornfield:

'Free' is not free from feelings, but free to feel each one and let it move on, unafraid of the movement of life… We can sense what feeling is at the center of each experience and open to it fully. This is a movement toward freedom.[6]

Kośas

Another framework for anchoring our awareness within the yoga tradition might be the *kośas,* which describe the human 'body' as consisting of five different layers (or sheaths), moving from that which is most gross and tangible (our physical body) to those that are more subtle (e.g., our spirit). These are:

- *annamaya kośa,* our physical body

- *prāṇamaya kośa,* our subtle energetic body (including the circulation systems governing our vital energy/*prāṇa,* blood, lymph etc.).

- *manomaya kośa,* our thoughts and emotions

- *vijñānamaya kośa,* our higher discerning/intuitive wisdom

- *ānandamaya kośa,* our 'bliss' body, the most subtle, spiritual layer where we feel connected to our true nature, that of peace, love, joy, sensing our inherent connection with all beings.

In bringing a mindful attention to these different layers of our being, we can consider how connected and caring we are towards each. As well as bringing attention to our body, breath and heart/mind, do we tune into and respond to our intuitive wisdom? Do we notice and access things that stimulate feelings of peace, joy and belonging?

As we become more intimate with all of these layers, we notice how intrinsically interlinked they are. We might recognize how the anxiety of our day has fed into our breath quickening and our body fidgeting; how a day of inactivity has left our mind grumpy, body achy and not knowing what we are needing; how sitting tall and open in a compassion meditation has softened our breath and lifted our spirits.

Our practice becomes a space where we can intentionally use this inherent connection to create positive changes. If life is feeling uncertain and changeable, we can tune into the sensation of our feet firmly rooted in Mountain Pose to cultivate feelings of steadiness and stability in our mind. If we are feeling small and lacking in confidence, we might take up space in Warrior 2, tapping into feelings of inner strength and spaciousness, letting them feed into our spirit.

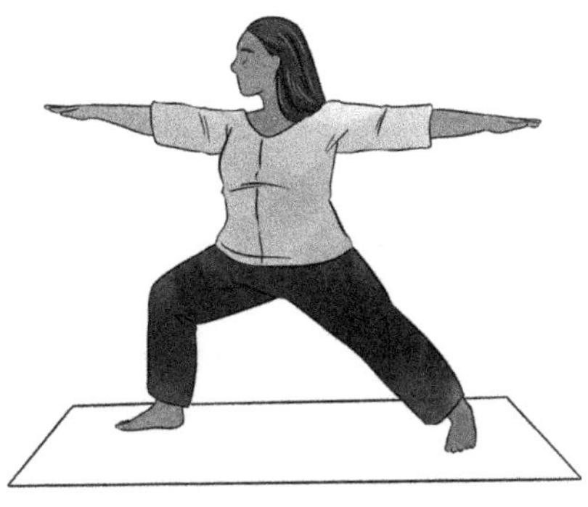

Warrior 2

Attitudes of mindful awareness

As we have seen, mindfulness isn't simply about *paying* attention, but about *how* we pay attention. In *Full Catastrophe Living*[7] Jon Kabat-Zinn outlines what he considers to be the key attitudes of mindful awareness. I find these a useful framework in my life, practice and teaching. We will explore what they are here and return to them in Section 3 to consider how we can guide our students towards them when teaching.

We can think of these attitudes like the lenses that opticians use to assess our vision. In any given moment, we might ask ourselves which lens we are looking through. Is it one that is helping or hindering our clear vision? Is it one that is moving us closer or further from feelings of peace and balance? Is it helping us to respond from a place of clarity and wise discernment?

It is important to see these not as qualities we are trying to perfect, nor judge ourselves harshly when we find them lacking. Rather, they are qualities we practise moving *towards*, inquiring whether we could bring in 'a little more' patience, kindness, openness or 'soften slightly' the judgements and demands that we so frequently place on ourselves.

You will notice that while many are similar in intention, they also have subtle nuances.

Beginner's mind

When we encounter something familiar, our tendency is to zone out from the detail, we find ourselves going through the motions, operating on auto-pilot without paying attention. A beginner's mind reminds us of the power of meeting life with child-like eyes, as if seeing something for the first time. It helps us remain open and curious, tuning into how things are, rather than how we expect or imagine them to be.

Within our yoga practice, this helps us to meet ourselves afresh despite having taken practices many, many times. It deepens our interest and engagement as we pay close attention to things that normally lie beneath our awareness (sensations in our body, the flow of our breath). It reminds us to make sure that our practice meets us where we are (not who we were yesterday or wish we were today), so that if we are tired or vibrant, we can adapt our practice accordingly.

Non-judgement

Our minds are eager to categorize experiences, deeming things 'good', 'bad', 'wanted', 'unwanted', 'right' or 'wrong'. Doing so impacts both the quality of attention we offer our experience and how we respond to it. Our brains are wired to respond differently depending on the 'feeling tone' (*vedana*) of an experience, whether pleasant, unpleasant or neutral. We naturally desire and move towards that which is deemed 'pleasant' (e.g., tasty food and warm shelter); are averse to and pull away from that which is deemed 'unpleasant' (e.g., a tiger); and dismiss or ignore that which is deemed neutral (and, therefore, doesn't warrant attention). While this makes sense from a survival perspective, in our modern lives it can lead to constantly striving for pleasing experiences, pushing away unpleasant ones and missing the beauty in the habitual.

These tendencies of mind form two of the *kleśas*. Patañjali highlights how our tendencies to cling to that which we desire (*rāga*) and pull away from that which is unpleasant (*dveṣa*) disrupts our peace of mind as we are buffeted around in a constant push/pull with life rather than navigating it skilfully or peacefully.

Judgements will naturally arise in our practice, but when we notice them (e.g., that touching the floor is 'good', my busy mind is 'bad', observing the breath is 'boring'), we practise softening them, acknowledging they are there without needing to believe in them. In my own experience, this can create such a shift in our practice, cultivating greater equanimity, which we will explore later.

Non-striving

Few of us come to practice with the hope of feeling the same at the end. It is our desire to feel 'better' that often draws us towards it. Neither desires nor goals are inherently bad, but we can sense when they are helpful or not. When our intention is dominated by striving, by wanting things to be a certain way, we often increase rather than lessen tension. It creates a push/pull within our practice; a pushing up against how things are; a striving towards how we wish things could be, like swimming against the tide, expending vast effort while being drawn further from the peace that we seek.

When in striving mode, our goal can be the driving force of our actions. With our gaze so fixed on a desired future state we risk missing what is before our eyes. Even when we do pay attention to the moment before us, it is only to assess our progress against a preferred state. This can lead to us bypassing messages our body is giving, which can increase our likelihood of injury. Goals have a habit of shifting; when one is attained, another brighter, glossier one often rises over the horizon, and before we know it, we are forever chasing an elusive happiness that is just out of reach.

In practising non-striving, our impetus for practice is more to open to what is here rather than to try to get somewhere. In doing so we reduce tendencies of pushing towards perfection. We see that the journey and the lessons we learn along the way are more valuable than a destination. It reminds us to listen to the wisdom of our body rather than being hijacked by the desires of our minds. It enables us to find greater contentment and gratitude for where we are, which can be life changing.

Acceptance

Acceptance can sometimes be misconstrued as passive resignation that this is how things are and we should simply endure it. This isn't the case and offers no agency for care or positive change (both personally and collectively). Acceptance, however, is about acknowledging rather than denying the reality of our lives. When our experience is painful, acceptance asks us to stay open and curious towards it, taking time to tenderly explore our experience (rather than numbing ourselves from it or leaping into action to immediately fix or change it). If our experience is positive or joyful, it allows us to notice and savour it.

By cultivating acceptance in our practice, we acknowledge our physical capabilities and limitations, we create space for the emotional states that arise without feeling they define the quality of our practice. As we learn to stay present to the feelings of a tight hamstring or the sadness held in our chest, we learn that we can be and breathe with it, rather than ignoring, denying or inflating it. Under these calmer conditions we can learn and grow from our experiences rather than feeling stuck in or destabilized by them. In offering the space to see clearly, we gain insights that help us discern what response is needed. We might think of the Serenity Prayer which offers: 'God grant me the serenity to accept the things I cannot change; courage to change the things I can; and wisdom to know the difference.'

Ironically, it is often in our allowing and accepting that things shift; the discomfort may still be there, but we have changed our relationship towards it, holding it more tenderly and reducing the suffering we add to it. In the words of Carl Rogers: 'The curious paradox is that when I accept myself just as I am, then I can change.'[8]

Letting go

Cultivating qualities of both acceptance and letting go may seem contradictory. But letting go is less about pushing things away and more about lessening our attachment to things needing to be a certain way. Life is inherently unpredictable and full of change; peace can be found when we acknowledge this, enabling us to 'go with the flow' rather than holding tightly onto how we wish things would be. We might think of letting go of the 'shoulds', the demands, the expectations we so often place on ourselves.

We can sense letting go on numerous levels: of tensions stored in the body, unhelpful default narratives in our minds, defensive knots around our hearts, all of which keep us in a more contracted, confined state. We learn to hold less tightly to our ego (our sense of 'I', 'me', 'mine') so that we are less defined by experience or protectively defending our sense of identity.

When letting go feels too scary or an impossible task, I like to reframe it as softening our grip. It is hard to let go of unhelpful conditioning and habits that have built over many years, but, little by little, we can learn to soften their edges, offering more breathing space around them.

Patience

In an age of high-speed and quick fixes, it is understandable that many people move fast and desire instant results. Life, however, can be complex, and creating sustainable change is a gradual process. It requires both presence and patience to keep moving forward, particularly given that 'progress' rarely follows a linear path.

Minds will wander, bodies will age and change. Life will bring with it joys and challenges. Patience offers us a gentle perseverance to stay on the path when we feel disheartened or frustrated. Patience helps us to soften comparisons and stop striving towards perfection.

In cultivating patience in our yoga practice, we are invited to slow down, understanding that we notice and learn more when we stop rushing through life. We practise patiently meeting ourselves, understanding that peace isn't found when we push or force, but when we create the conditions for things to unfold in their own time. In the words of Jack Kornfield: 'Our body, heart and spirit know how to give birth, to open naturally, like the petals of a flower. We need not tear at the petals nor force the flower. We must simply stay planted and present.'[9]

Trust

So often, we look towards external sources to determine what is 'right', 'wrong', 'good' or 'bad'. We seek answers from society, our peers, our teachers, handing over agency to others rather than trusting the wisdom that lies deep within ourselves.

When our minds are noisy with thoughts, it can be hard to connect to our more intuitive wisdom. The more disconnected we are from our bodies, the less we pick up its signals when something *feels* right or *feels* wrong for us. Creating the conditions in which we can listen to and respond to our 'inner teacher', our intuition, is important in guiding us forward in life in a way that feels true to ourselves. Many of us need to strengthen our capacity to listen and respond to this layer of our being (*vijñānamaya kośa* – the wisdom sheath).

When we are in a heightened emotional state, it can be hard to access our intuition because the fear-based part of our mind is eager to keep us safe and alert to danger. As our nervous system calms and our mental chatter quietens, it becomes easier to hear that intuitive part of ourselves. Often during a practice, an answer will suddenly appear to things that we have been ruminating over before a class. It is why we often have our 'Aha' moments on holiday or when relaxing in the bath.

Our yoga practice offers an opportunity to connect with, listen to and respond to our intuitive wisdom. In doing so we become more attuned to the messages offered by the body when it is saying 'yes' or 'no'. We can more wisely discern whether something is helpful or harmful, when we should move forward, pull back, be active or take rest. Patañjali acknowledges that one path doesn't fit all, that it is about seeking the path that fits the individual. As we deepen our capacity to listen to and trust in our personal truth within our practice, we strengthen our capacity to follow it in our wider lives.

We might also think of trust as having faith in the process of our practice, so that we remember to persevere when times are difficult or our practice seems to plateau.

Accessing equanimity

Equanimity is about meeting of the ups and downs of life with a calm composure. We have seen how life consists of varying feeling tones (pleasant, unpleasant and neutral). Equanimity reminds us that the nature of life is one of flux and change, it includes moments of joy and pain as well as aspects that seem bland or undramatic. In cultivating equanimity we practise bringing a kind, curious, balanced attention to it all. We recognize that the nature of worldly things (in both our inner and outer worlds) is one of impermanence.

We cultivate equanimity within our yoga practice as we learn to open to that which feels pleasant (e.g., a moment of peace in *Śavāsana*) without feeling dismayed when it comes to an end; remain curious towards that which is neutral (e.g., the flow of our breath) and normally slips beneath our awareness; and learn to hold unpleasant experiences (e.g., a strong sensation as we meet our edge of stretch) in a balanced awareness, neither distracting ourselves nor inflating it via the stories layered onto it (e.g., 'This is horrible', 'I am awful at yoga').

The Mountain Meditation (see Section 2) is a beautiful practice to connect us to a quality of equanimity amid the shifting nature of life's experiences.

Gratitude

If you've ever thought you were a 'glass half empty' person, you might be pleased to understand that our brains have an inbuilt negativity bias. Again, this makes sense from a survival perspective, but doesn't steer us towards happiness. If we were walking through a scene consisting of many pleasant things (flowers, birds, sunshine), neutral things (the concrete path) and one unpleasant thing (an angry person), it is understandable that our brain would lock hold of the angry person over the beautiful flowers as it perceives it as a threat. In our lives today, this negativity bias plays out in numerous ways, meaning that we can be more fixated on what we don't know than what we do, or on the person who appeared to not enjoy our class over the many who said they did.

The neuroscientist and meditation teacher Rick Hanson offers a helpful analogy for this: that negative experiences stick in our neurology in milliseconds like Velcro, while positive experiences, unless we offer them our prolonged attention (he suggests 5–20 seconds) slip off like Teflon.[10]

Mindfulness enables us to notice and counterbalance this natural bias, so that when we experience something positive, we take time to not only notice, but to savour and feel grateful for it, enabling it to embed in our neurology, therefore, offering us a more balanced and accurate (and often more optimistic) perspective on our lives.

Within our yoga practice, we can choose to consciously tune into and celebrate our capabilities rather than focus solely on perceived deficiencies. We can rest our attention for prolonged periods on aspects of our experience that feel positive (e.g., where we sense qualities of strength, support, ease, peace or vitality).

It is worth noting that we consciously open to that which is good not to distract ourselves from life's difficulties, but rather to see our lives from a more accurate perspective, less distorted by our negativity bias; doing so enables us to feel gratitude for what we *have* rather focusing solely on what we lack.

Noticing habitual patterns

As we begin to see ourselves more clearly, we notice habitual patterns that play out both in our lives and practice. In yoga these are known as *saṃskāras*, we might think of them as well-worn paths that play out in our bodies, hearts and minds that deepen with regular repetition.

They might present as patterns of tension or weakness in the body, patterns of ease or restriction in the breath, patterns of peace or preoccupation in the mind, patterns of joy or fear in the heart. We become aware of their causes and impact (e.g., when I sit at my computer all day my posture rounds and it creates backache) as well as how inherently interlinked the different layers of our being are.

We begin to see how patterns that play out in our wider lives meet us on the mat. Patterns of perfectionism, striving, fear or lack of confidence can be seen in how we hold and move our bodies, whether forever pushing beyond what is sustainable, needing to take the hardest option, forever backing away from our edge or denying ourselves rest. Our practice offers space to cultivate new, more supportive *saṃskāras* (e.g., improved posture, breathing, cultivating qualities of mindful awareness), which through regular repetition on the mat begin to spill into the fabric of our everyday lives.

In bringing these often unconscious habits to our conscious awareness, we notice which move us closer towards peace and wellbeing (*saṃyoga*) and practice cultivating them, as well as which are damaging and detrimental to it (*viyoga*) and practice reducing them. We become aware of what lights us up, what pushes our buttons, what makes us feel whole and connected or dull and scattered. This helps us sense how and when we have fallen off balance and what is required to guide us back towards it.

We see that traits that we consider 'just the way I am' aren't so fixed and solid; while they may have strengthened over years of repetition, new pathways can be cultivated. Even over a short period of practice we can sense the shift from arriving feeling contracted, distracted and disconnected to leaving feeling more at ease, focused and whole. Over a longer period of practice we might notice ourselves becoming less reactive, more open, stronger, more focused or calm. Of course, life still happens, but we become more able to self-regulate when needed.

Navigating pain and difficulty

As we meet life with greater awareness, we open not only to what is joyful and pleasing, but also that which is painful and challenging. This is the nature of life. It is here that mindfulness links with compassion. Mindfulness enables us to *notice* when pain is present (whether our own or another's). It reminds us to remain open to and curious about it (rather than pulling away from or feeling overwhelmed by it). It helps us to clearly see the causes and conditions contributing to it. Compassion offers a way of skilfully *responding* to it, meeting it with care and tenderness, offering a supportive presence and lessening the suffering while in the midst of it.

Pain is a natural part of being human, physically, mentally and emotionally. While marketing machines might make us feel that if we had, did or achieved 'enough' we could banish it, the truth is that peace is found when we skilfully navigate it.

While yoga can draw us closer towards our inherent lightness, the path involves gently opening to our darkness, the parts of ourselves that we might hide from – our tight corners and uncomfortable feelings. Our lightness comes from seeing and reducing that which blocks it, rather than bypassing shadows that inevitably cross it.

While pain is an inevitable aspect of life – we experience pleasure and pain, love and loss, joy and sorrow – suffering is considered optional. The Buddha beautifully illustrates the difference between pain and suffering in his analogy of the first and second arrows. He asked his disciples if they would feel pain if they were struck by an arrow, to which they agreed 'yes'. He then asked if they would feel more pain if they were struck by a second arrow, to which they understandably agreed 'yes'.

The Buddha shared that, in life, pain is like the first arrow. We didn't ask to be struck by an arrow and yet it has struck; we feel pain, that is inevitable. But suffering is found in the second arrow: the layers of judgements or narratives that we fire at ourselves (or others) in response to the first. We might think of accidentally stubbing our toe as being the first arrow, while the narratives of 'you're such an idiot', 'this has ruined my day', 'who put that there, no one cares about me' as being the second. While the first is inevitable and potentially short lived, our secondary arrows can add fuel to the fire, making our suffering burn brighter for longer.

It can be helpful to understand that our brain's survival focus means that we are hard-wired to pull away from pain. This makes sense when pulling our hand away from a fire or running away from the tiger, but it doesn't help us explore, tend to or grow from discomfort that isn't life threatening.

We might sense in ourselves how difficult it is to 'be' with pain, to open to it and feel it. Understandably we fall into patterns of distracting or numbing ourselves from it or battling to fix it, often expending vast amounts of energy doing so without necessarily alleviating it (often creating additional layers on top of it).

Mindfulness invites us to approach pain differently, softening our resistance and gently turning towards it, leaning in rather than pulling away, holding it in a steady, spacious, kind container so that we can objectively explore rather than feel so overwhelmed by it. In doing so we sense that, while pain may not feel pleasant, it often has something to teach us; that rather than it being a fixed, solid entity, it too is subject to changes and shifts; that while it is a part of our experience, we don't need to be defined by it. It allows us to find greater acceptance for the first arrow, while noticing and lessening the secondary arrows that we fire on top of it.

Our ability to heal, grow and thrive requires us to open to the whole of ourselves, including pain and discomfort. We build resilience when we develop our capacity to listen to and learn from life's challenges rather than feeling defined or controlled by them. This increases what Dan Siegel terms our 'window of tolerance',[11] our ability to open to the broad range of life's experiences with greater equanimity. In doing so, we are reminded that while we can't always change what life throws at us, we can change how we respond to it. This can enable us to feel more resourced, resilient and empowered within life's challenges. We begin to sense that peace isn't reliant on life being as we wish it, but rather in our ability to ride the ups and downs mindfully and compassionately. In the words of Jon Kabat-Zinn: 'You can't stop the waves but you can learn to surf.'[12]

Our yoga practice can provide a useful training ground for navigating pain and difficulty. When we experience discomfort, do we judge ourselves for it or can we be compassionate towards it? Each time we meet our 'edge' in a pose, we have an opportunity to practise gently being with that which is less than comfortable. That said, being gentle doesn't mean avoiding challenges. Our practice offers us space to explore both our limits *and* our capabilities which can include noticing our relationship to challenges. As we meet our edge of comfort (which can be felt emotionally as much as physically), do we tend to pull away, or push and force beyond it? With mindful awareness we learn to stay open to and respectfully explore it. While many of us find it easier to feel the discomfort of a tight hamstring than a hurting heart, practising with the former can provide useful training for the latter.

We might recognize that 'difficult', 'discomfort' and 'challenging' can take different forms. For some, stillness is more uncomfortable than movement, softening more challenging than a handstand.

Whether working with our own or a client's pain, we are required to work wisely and sensitively. At times pain offers clear messages that require action (whether to pull away or seek support), at others it can be transformative to simply offer it a caring, listening presence, softening the secondary suffering that we add to it. At other times, leaning towards our pain may simply be too overwhelming (which is neither helpful nor healing) and the most compassionate action might be to take practices that soothe and stabilize us while in the midst of it.

Chapter 2

WHAT IS COMPASSION?

As we have seen mindfulness and compassion are intrinsically inter-linked. While mindfulness supports us in seeing ourselves more clearly, learning to hold difficult feelings in a balanced, caring attention, compassion brings with it a quality of action, enabling us to tend to and lessen (rather than ignore or inflate) it. In the words of Tara Brach:

> The two parts of genuine acceptance – seeing clearly and holding our experience with compassion – are as interdependent as the two wings of a great bird. Together they enable us to fly and be free.[1]

'Compassion' comes from the Latin roots 'com' (with) and 'pati' (to suffer), so can be thought of as the willingness to 'suffer with'. This doesn't mean taking on the suffering of another, but rather being a supportive presence while either we or others move through it. Empathy is an integral element of compassion; it enables us to recognize, feel and relate to the pain of another, which in turn stimulates compassion, a desire to take action to alleviate it. In the words of Paul Gilbert: 'Compassion can be defined as behaviour that aims to nurture, look after, teach, guide, mentor, soothe, protect, offer feelings of acceptance and belonging – in order to benefit another person'.[2]

Feelings of care, kindness and belonging are essential to our wellbeing. When we find or perceive ourselves as separated or ostracized from our 'group', we inevitably feel vulnerable. From a survival perspective, being separated from our pack or tribe would place us in greater danger. As such, our nervous system would likely move into a threat response (e.g., the sympathetic nervous system taking us into fight/flight mode, or the dorsal vagal aspect of the parasympathetic nervous system taking us into the freeze response). Here, systems relating to long-term health and wellbeing are suppressed as our energy is shunted towards our survival (e.g., fighting, fleeing or freezing).

In giving and receiving care and kindness, we sense ourselves as a part of a caring community, which can promote feelings of safety in our 'belonging'. Acts of kindness (e.g., caring words, touch, actions) stimulate oxytocin, often known as the 'love hormone', that promotes feelings of connection, safety and belonging, which in turn help us to feel calm. As Paul Gilbert writes in *Mindful Compassion,* 'our brains are set up to be *calmed down in the face of kindness*'.[3] In these conditions, we move into the ventral vagal aspect of our parasympathetic nervous system, which promotes feelings of calm. It is in these calmer conditions that our threat response is calmed. Here, psychological and physiological systems that benefit our long-term health and wellbeing (rather than short term survival) work optimally (e.g., social engagement, digestion, reproduction, circulation, respiration, our immune system).

Our yoga practice offers space to notice our relationship towards ourselves and others and steer us towards more compassionate connections. We will explore practical ways of applying this within our yoga teaching in Section 3, but for now let's explore what we mean by *self*-compassion.

Self-compassion

Compassion can be extended outwardly towards others or inwardly towards ourselves; however, many of us find it easy to do the former, and struggle with the latter. When a friend or a loved one experiences pain or difficulty, our immediate response is often to offer a kind, listening ear, to be gentle and understanding with them and see how we can best support them. The tone of our response serves to calm and soothe them, offering a sense of perspective, signalling connection.

When it comes to ourselves, however, our manner often contrasts significantly. Our pain or difficulty is sometimes interpreted as a sign of inadequacy or failing, and we then respond to it more harshly and judgementally, dismissing our need to be soothed and cared for. Inevitably, this increases feelings of isolation and separation which only feed our stress and suffering.

The closest, most important and impactful relationship we will ever have is the one with ourselves, but without gentle, persistent effort, it is often overlooked and undervalued. While marketing machines may feed us messages that if only we were 'smarter', 'richer', 'thinner', 'curvier' *then* we could love ourselves, self-compassion reminds us that we can do so right here, right now, in all our imperfect humanness. Our conditioning may throw up resistance (perceiving it as silly, selfish, self-indulgent, arrogant or weak); therefore, self-compassion is something that many of us need to consciously practice.

In her book *Self-Compassion*, Kristin Neff, outlines what she considers to be the core components of self-compassion: mindfulness, common humanity and self-kindness.[4] Let's explore them here in the context of meeting ourselves in moments of pain or difficulty.

Mindfulness

We've explored mindfulness previously in detail, but in the context of suffering it enables us to acknowledge and open to painful feelings; noticing our habitual responses towards them (whether to deny, try to fix or inflate them); and offers the conditions to gently explore them in how they play out within us, through body, mind and heart (e.g., physical sensations, thoughts and emotions).

Common humanity

Common humanity reminds us that pain and difficulty are a natural and inevitable part of life. While their nature and circumstances will vary, their presence is universal. Being human involves losses and knocks; we age, we decay, we make mistakes. Even when our behaviours appear unwise or unhelpful, we might acknowledge that they are often steered by unconscious forces which make them more understandable. That's not to say we don't take responsibility for our choices but rather lessen tendencies of self-loathing and shaming, the secondary arrows that often keep us small and stuck, rather than learning and growing from our experiences. Seen in this context, the pain we inevitably experience, as well as our perceived flaws and challenges, offer points of *connection* with others rather than aspects that alienate and distances us. Words I love, suggested by Judith Hanson Lasater (and I use them often in my life and teaching), are: 'How very human of me!'.

Self-kindness

Something I recognize in myself and see in others is how very hard we can be on ourselves. While some of the pain we experience comes from what life throws at us, much of it comes from what we throw at ourselves.

In cultivating self-kindness, we learn to treat ourselves as we would a dear friend, meeting ourselves with care and tenderness. This can involve the way that we speak to ourselves (our tone of voice, the words we say to ourselves), how we respond through our actions (whether offering conditions of kindness and care, withholding them or punishing ourselves).

Self-soothing

As we learn to become a more compassionate companion towards ourselves, we develop our capacity to soothe ourselves in difficult times. This is an essential element in being able to self-regulate after difficult experiences. Paul Gilbert talks of us having three emotional regulation systems:[5]

- *Drive and resource seeking system,* which motivates and activates us to meeting our essential survival needs (e.g., seeking food, shelter, sexual partners).

- *Threat and self-protection system,* which either activates (fight/flight) or inhibits (freeze) our actions to keep us safe and protected from threat.

- *Soothing and affiliation system,* which supports our need for safety, care and connection, and leads to us feeling calm and content.

When I explore these drives with clients, there is often agreement that they spend a lot of time in the 'drive and resource seeking' system (which, when out of balance, can feed into patterns of overly striving and wanting) and the 'threat and self-protect' system (which, when out of balance, can feed into patterns of anxiety or depression), but hadn't considered the importance of prioritizing and nourishing the 'soothing and affiliation' system where we feel a sense of contentment, safety and belonging.

While many of us are familiar with seeking signals of safety, connection, worth and belonging from external sources (e.g., feeling settled and soothed when on the receiving end of caring words and actions from others), we are often less familiar with offering the same towards ourselves.

In Section 3 we will explore practical ways to support students in:

- meeting themselves mindfully

- connecting with their common humanity, sensing that they are a part of a caring, collective community rather than in competition, with themselves or others

- cultivating kindness through the way they approach themselves

- incorporating self-soothing, through words and actions.

I would encourage you to explore these in your own life and practice.

Relief, resistance and revelations

As someone who grew up with the words 'must have more self-confidence' on most school reports, learning about self-compassion (rather than self-esteem or self-confidence) felt a revelation. In my younger years, the idea of 'loving myself' seemed to suggest that I should think myself utterly brilliant, which felt both untrue and arrogant. On days when life felt challenging, qualities of self-confidence and self-esteem felt out of reach.

When I learnt about self-compassion, what resonated with me most was that it wasn't asking me to strive towards excellence, nor present as super confident, but to simply show up to the reality of my life (all the beautiful, messy and imperfect parts) and meet it with kindness rather than criticism. For me this was liberating. It helped to comfort me on difficult days and to see my quirks and mistakes as something that connects me to others, rather than failings that prevent me from belonging.

Over time, it helped me to feel calmer, happier, more resilient within life's wobbles and, funnily enough, more quietly confident.

It is understandable, however, that cultivating any new relationship with ourselves can be emotional or met with resistance. I remember the first time a teacher invited me to stroke my face in a caring manner; my body softened, my breath deepened and tears unexpectedly flowed as I sensed my ability to be my own caregiver while recognizing how long I had denied myself this.

Kindness and compassion are powerful and so must be approached with sensitivity. While often perceived as 'soft' or 'gentle' qualities, they require strength and courage to practice. It's not uncommon for feelings of grief or shame to surface as we recognize the secondary arrows we've been firing at ourselves. Offering compassion can involve softening the armour that we have protectively built around ourselves; while loosening it may feel a relief, it can also feel scary. Anything new can feel clunky or uncomfortable and it's understandable that we might feel resistance towards it. These are all normal responses which require respect and sensitivity to our individual histories and needs, taking things slowly, adapting the pace and practices accordingly.

Other common responses are feelings of frustration or failure when we struggle with a practice or our inner dialogue is uncompassionate. Again, 'progress' is rarely linear. I have been asked by students if, after all these years of practice, self-compassion is now my default mode. As much as I wish it were different, the answer is 'no' (the survival habits of my brain are still fit and strong). But as with anything, the more often we practise something, the more accessible it feels and the more strength it gains.

I remember a few years ago when I did something 'silly' and the words 'Argh you're such an idiot!' blasted out internally. I was surprised to discover another kinder voice quickly leaping to my defence with 'No, you're not sweetheart'. 'Ah', I thought, 'it *does* work!'.

But, of course, there are other times when I forget, noticing only when the impact is of doing so is coursing through my body, heart and mind. As we will explore more in Section 2, our inner critic (and its close companion, imposter syndrome) may be lifelong companions, but we can become more aware of them and build more compassionate companions to accompany them.

I feel it's important to stress that self-compassion doesn't ask us to be fully self-reliant in meeting our support needs. Sometimes, the most self-compassionate thing we can do is reach out for support from others. There will be times when it's harder to access these tools – perhaps when we are strongly triggered or depleted – and we benefit from an external source, whether a friend, colleague or mentor/supervisor, to help guide us back towards them. This is not failing; it is wise, compassionate action. Self-compassion means that we can be a part of our personal support network, but not the sole member.

Self-compassion is something that we practise, not aim to perfect. We don't succeed when we are saintly beings, but in the small moments when we remember to ask ourselves: 'Could I bring a little more kindness towards this?'. Practising on days when life is smooth helps us to access it when it feels rocky.

Widening our circle of caring

Cultivating self-compassion is far from selfish. The more we offer, 'How very human of me!' and respond with kindness, the more we can acknowledge, 'How very human of *you*!' and do the same. Rather than our hearts opening only to those who we know well, or feel deserve it, we widen our circle of caring to those who we don't know well or find challenging (e.g., the new student in our class or the one who arrives late and hurriedly slams down their mat!), understanding that each of us has difficulties and complexities that lie beneath the surface.

The Loving Kindness meditation is a beautiful practice to support this (see Chapter 20), helping us sense our interconnectivity and shared humanness; enabling us to appreciate that even those whose behaviours we find difficult are often motivated from a place of seeking happiness, even if we disagree with how they try to achieve it. It doesn't mean that we need to like or condone their actions, but we can appreciate more fully the complexities and vulnerabilities of being human and how we are all guided by unconscious forces that shape our lived experience.

Over time, the distinction we place between 'me' and 'you', 'us' and 'them' softens, we recognize our deep connection with all beings and we broaden the range for which our heart opens. We understand that our own personal peace doesn't sit in isolation but rather is intrinsically interlinked with peace within our wider community, which then guides our actions.

Finding balance

It is human nature to fall out of balance. In Robin Wall Kimmerer's beautiful book *Braiding Sweetgrass,* she talks about the process of clearing and cleaning a pond and offers: 'Balance is not a passive resting place – it takes work, balancing the giving and the taking, the raking out and the putting in'[6] – words which echo our wider lives.

Balance is more of a dance than a destination; a dance between giving and receiving, doing and resting, actively shaping and gracefully accepting. Just as we can't control the ecosystems of the pond, we can't always control the environment of our lives, but we can put in the work to create more balance within them.

Sometimes, it requires putting things back in (e.g., movement or rest, joy or caring connection); sometimes, it requires raking things out (unhelpful inner narratives, over activity, expectations and judgements). It is a dance that continues throughout our life; like a pond, it requires work, and our practice offers us the space to do this.

Many traditions recognize that peace and wellbeing are accessed when we are in a state of balance. In the Buddha's search for liberation, he recognized that peace wasn't to be found in hedonistic lifestyles of excess nor the self-denial and penance of the ascetics. The path beyond suffering was found in a 'middle way', a path of balance between extremes.

Within the yoga tradition, we see this reflected in the *guṇas*, qualities found in varying degrees in all matter (e.g., both our internal state of body, heart, mind and external objects).

- *Rajas* offers qualities of movement and activity, but when out of balance might be experienced as an inability to stop, a fidgety body or an anxious mind.

- *Tamas* offers qualities of steadiness and stillness, but when out of balance might be experiences in feeling lethargic, stuck or depressed.

- *Sattva* offers qualities of clarity, peace and harmony which we experience when we reduce excessive *rajas* and *tamas*. We might consider it a state of wellbeing and balance.

Like the pond, these qualities are in a constant state of flux and change, but by paying attention we can notice when they are in or out of balance and what will move us closer towards a more *sattvic* state.

While mindfulness helps us see how we have fallen out of balance, compassionate action steers us back towards it.

Chapter 3

MINDFUL, COMPASSIONATE YOGA

While mindful awareness and compassionate action lie at the heart of yoga, it is easy to practice with the absence of them. We might notice this in ourselves when we find ourselves on auto-pilot, going through the motions on the mat but lost in thought. We might sense this in our students as faces tense with frustration or hearts contract with inner criticism. Without careful attention, our practice can become yet another place in which we perpetuate our imbalances rather than notice and redress them. We need safe, supportive spaces that help us in remembering.

Becoming more intimate with ourselves is a courageous act, one that requires an open, tender heart rather than a fierce, gripping fist. With mindfulness and compassion at its centre, our yoga practice becomes a refuge, a place that holds us wherever we are, rather than another setting in which we feel we need to perform or prove our worth. Sometimes, we can create this container for ourselves; sometimes, we benefit from stepping into a caring container created by another teacher.

Our practice offers space for reconnection, to notice what lies beneath the surface of the daily 'doing'; a space where the disparate parts of ourselves can be seen, felt, gathered and held. Being human is not a state of perfection, but often complex and sometimes messy. Our practice is a place to meet ourselves, not to escape or supersede our reality. It offers space to acknowledge and cultivate our strengths as well as meet our vulnerabilities; to gently progress rather than push for perfection. As we soften the expectations and demands that we so often place on ourselves we learn to open our hearts to however we are (rather than waiting until we become a 'better' version of ourselves).

We are all unique and one size does not fit all. When practising mindfully, our practice is something we shape around our needs, rather than mould ourselves into how we think we should be. The nature of our practice will naturally change, as we do in life, but the quality and benefits of our practice are neither enhanced nor limited by our age, size or level of fitness or flexibility.

In slowing down our pace in our practice, we dial up our awareness. Rather than rushing through life, we open to it. Slowness guides us towards stillness, space to be and rest. As nervous systems balance, bodies soften, hearts open and mental chatter quietens, we rest in awareness, observing the life that moves through us without feeling so entangled in it.

In seeing how and where we have fallen out of balance, we begin to recognize how very human this is. Rather than getting lost in layers of self-criticism, we can access practices that guide us back towards it. We notice how our capacity for self-regulation isn't confined to the mat but can be incorporated into our daily lives.

As our mind quietens, our intuition can be more easily heard. In offering space to listen and respond to the insights that arise, we are steered towards a path that feels more authentic and aligned with the way we want to be living. We may feel a sense of wholeness and less scattered, in touch with a more authentic version of ourselves, less identified with the roles that life demands of us. Feelings of belonging deepen, as we sense our inherent connection to one another.

While our practice on the mat provides a training ground for our hearts and minds to be more open and present, the fruits of our practice play out in the quality of our actions and interactions in our everyday lives. All of this deepens our capacity to move through life with greater clarity, stability, peace and sustainability. We do so not just for our personal benefit, but for wider world and the communities we share it with, sensing our intrinsic connectivity.

SUPPORTING OURSELVES AS TEACHERS

'Mindfulness not only makes it possible to survey our inner landscape with compassion and curiosity but can also actively steer us in the right direction for self-care.'[1]

Bessel Van Der Kolk

Overview

The first stage in embedding any new learning into our teaching is to incorporate it into our own practice. By taking time to explore and absorb our own experience of mindfulness and compassion, our teaching of it comes from an embodied 'knowing' rather than purely an intellectual understanding. It helps us recognize and appreciate both the benefits and challenges our students may experience as they practice. When I consider teachers who most resonate with me, it is as much, if not more, about how they embody the teachings as the words they say. It is felt in how they hold themselves and the space, interact with students and share practices. We sense when someone's teaching comes not just from the head but from the heart.

This section explores ways of incorporating mindfulness and compassion within your own life and teaching. If these concepts are new to you, I would highly recommend attending a teacher-led mindfulness course over a period of weeks to deepen your practice.

In the first part of this section, we will consider our personal practice. You might like to reach for a journal as you do so to jot down insights and reflections that arise. The latter part will consider how mindfulness and compassion steer us in the direction of self-care, supporting our wellbeing and sustainability within our teaching.

My intention is that this section offers practical suggestions and space for exploration and reflection, enabling you to explore how mindfulness and compassion might support *your* wellbeing before we shift the focus to our students in Section 3.

—— *Chapter 4* ——

OUR PERSONAL PRACTICE

Let us remember Rumi's question: 'Do you pay regular visits to yourself?'

The nature of our practice and the type of visitor we are to it will inevitably vary. As we transition from student to teacher, we often sense a shift as our passion becomes our profession; what once felt personal and precious can become something we feel we *have* to do because we are a teacher rather than something we *choose* to do because we are human and it helps us feel better.

Like all relationships, as we move beyond the honeymoon phase, we experience ups and downs, moments of excitement and discovery, moments of stagnation and lack of inspiration. We age, we change, we discover new influences and trainings. There will be days when our practice feels a delight and others when we need discipline to draw us towards it. At any point in our journey, it can get sidelined by busyness or morphed into lesson planning. What is important is that we remain attentive to it, create space for it and offer ourselves compassion when we struggle to connect with it.

What I notice in myself is that if my practice comes from a sense of obligation, it becomes somewhat stale and dry, like the heart has been taken out of it. I begin to assess it against how it 'should' look given that I'm a teacher. With mindfulness and compassion at its centre, however, the 'shoulds' begin to lessen and possibilities open. It becomes more a space for self-care and self-exploration rather than self-improvement, a refuge to be drawn towards rather than an obligation to be dragged to.

Over the years, I've got better at meeting myself where I am and adapting my practice accordingly. There are days when it takes place on the mat or meditation cushion, (or a small stretch of carpet); others when it involves walking in nature, listening to the birds singing or lying in bed taking a Body Scan or doing *yoganidrā*. Some days, it centres on breathing and moving; on others, resting and sitting. There are days when I enjoy holding space for myself, and others when I need to feel held and guided by other teachers. Whatever shape it takes, it reminds me of the power of these practices, that simple things, when undertaken with awareness, can create significant shifts.

In incorporating the attitudes of mindful awareness within our yoga practice, we remember to meet ourselves with kind, curious eyes. As we soften expectations and judgements, our practice can offer a safe space where sadness and playfulness are equally welcome, where movement and stillness, doing and being can find balance. At times, we might feel steady and strong enough to tend to difficult feelings; at others, we may need to build our store of care and compassion before being ready for it.

One of my yoga therapy clients, also a yoga teacher, was feeling depleted and overwhelmed due to personal and professional challenges. On further exploration, she noted that she didn't have the energy to explore the difficult feelings that lurked beneath her busyness, and this made her resistant to her yoga practice. We explored reframing her practice as a place of refuge in which she could tenderly nourish, soothe and steady herself during this difficult period. She found this to be transformative. We acknowledged that her practice could still be a space to tend to difficult feelings but only when she felt resourced and resilient enough for it.

I've often heard teachers admitting to feeling ashamed that they are not doing 'enough' or aren't as 'disciplined' as they feel they 'should' be regarding their practice. Yet when exploring yoga in its broader context, off that mat, a different story is presented. While it is essential that we offer ourselves time outside of our daily tasks to practice what we teach, we can also appreciate the varying shapes our practice can take.

Here again, the *kośas* model may feel useful, reminding us to consider how we are tending to the different layers of ourselves, both on and off the mat. We might ask:

- *Annamaya kośa:* How am I caring for my body?

- *Prāṇamaya kośa:* How am I tending to my vital energy?

- *Manomaya kośa:* How am I caring for my mental and emotional health?

- *Vijñānamaya kośa:* How am I listening and responding to my intuition?

- *Ānandamaya kośa:* How am I nourishing my spirit, my sense of love, peace, connection and joy?

Considering this final, most subtle layer helps us appreciate that accessing that which nourishes our spirit is as important to our wellbeing as the nutritional content of the food we eat. For those of us prone to postponing the 'nice stuff' until the to-do list is done (which, let's face it, never happens!), this can help us to reframe and prioritize them as a part of our daily practice .

Section 3 offers practical ways of incorporating mindfulness and compassion into our teaching, and you may find these useful to explore within your own practice also.

REFLECTIONS

Take a moment to consider your relationship with your personal practice.

- Does it feel a supportive space to meet yourself, to offer yourself care and nourishment?

- Do you feel pressure or judgements regarding how it 'should' look as a teacher?

- Does your practice allow for balance between doing and being, shaping and allowing, activity and stillness?

- How does your practice adapt to meet your varying needs?

- Does meditation form a regular part of your practice?

> – Can you acknowledge and celebrate ways that your practice spills into your daily life?
>
> – Are there attitudes of mindful awareness that you feel you would benefit from exploring more deeply within your practice?

Tending to ourselves

Teaching yoga can be inspiring and energizing. My heart often feels uplifted when teaching; watching students re-connecting to themselves, learning to befriend and tend to their bodies, calm their minds, open their hearts and create more balance in their lives.

But, as with any caregiving profession, teaching yoga can also be tiring. From the outside looking in, the role of the teacher can appear effortless and calm, but, like a gliding swan, there is a lot going on beneath the surface.

We often work alone, which can feel isolating. In addition to our direct teaching, there are many hours (often unpaid and less inspiring) involved in marketing, planning, travel and admin. I've often heard from teachers in training who were surprised to discover there is so much to consider, manage and navigate while calmly holding space for others to practice.

If teaching is our sole source of revenue, there can be financial stresses with insecure and fluctuating incomes, no holiday or sick pay. Social media can skew our perception so that we feel lost in a sea of competition rather than a valuable member of a community of teachers. Our brain's negativity bias can allow inner critics to run riot. The realities and daily demands of earning a living can make it difficult to prioritize our own wellbeing. Burn out is common.

Highly selective imagery presented by social media can often feed into the misconception that the life of a yoga teacher is idyllic. I've seen videos online depicting 'a day in the life of a yoga teacher' which present stress-free days of self-practice, smoothie drinking, teaching serenely calm students, reading spiritual books before a spot of paddleboarding. While these teachers may be the lucky ones, I imagine it doesn't reflect the reality for many of us. Where is the sinking feeling when only one person shows up for class or when on hands and knees wiping the floor because the cleaner was late in leaving? Where is the internet crashing moments before an online workshop or the sound of children arguing before muting? These are often the realities that we are also navigating.

The experience of being taught is very different from teaching. As professionals, we often invest significantly in developing skills to best support our students, yet it is equally important that we set aside time to consider how to best support ourselves. Doing the work we love requires us to be resourced. As the saying goes, 'You can't pour from an empty cup'.

Tending to ourselves is far from selfish. The more we prioritize holding space for ourselves, the more confident we become in holding space for others. The more we learn to offer ourselves care and nourishment, the more grounded and present we are likely to feel when teaching. The more we practise self-compassion, the less our inner critic rules the show; all of which benefits not just ourselves but also our students. In the words of Jack Kornfield: 'If we are to bring light and wisdom and compassion into this world, we must first begin with ourselves'.[1]

Chapter 5

WHAT IS SELF-CARE?

Take a moment to consider what self-care means to you. Elements that lie at the heart of it might be:

- making our actions caring towards ourselves

- looking after our personal wellbeing

- checking that what we ask of ourselves is realistic

- meeting ourselves with loving kindness (being patient and understanding rather than harsh and self-critical)

- prioritizing ourselves along with the roles we play in this world for others (e.g., family, students, employers)

- offering ourselves rest, nourishment and nurturing

- listening to our needs and learning to express and respond to them.

For some, the concept of self-care can seem vague, or else tied up with notions of spa days or bubble baths. As lovely as these can be, self-care stretches far beyond this. Sometimes, it involves taking rest or seeking joy; sometimes, it involves saying 'no' or being clear and confident in our boundaries; it can include ensuring that our fees enable us to be sick, take holidays or have a pension to care for ourselves in old age. It can involve creating supportive communities where we feel seen, safe, held and heard. Rather than being soft or fluffy as it can sometimes be perceived, it is a courageous commitment to ensuring that our own needs aren't sidelined.

It can be about creating small, impactful changes that don't need to be costly.

> **REFLECTION**
>
> – In what ways do you prioritize self-care within your life and teaching?

Self-care or self-improvement?

Although self-care and self-improvement seem similar, their *impact* is quite different. When self-improvement is the driving force, our actions may stem from a sense of lacking, of not being good enough, needing fixing or, the other end of the spectrum, being better than everyone else. With this kind of motivation, our actions or practice can feel more effortful. Judgements more commonly arise while assessing ourselves for signs of progress and improvement, often in comparison to others.

When self-care is our driving force, our heart may feel more open to how we are, rather than focused on how we would like ourselves to be. It can offer more space for listening rather than needing to immediately leap into action to change things. It can feel empowering to recognize that we can offer ourselves care, regardless of the condition we find ourselves in.

Exploring barriers to self-care

Many of us recognize the benefits of self-care but struggle to prioritize it. Shining a light on our barriers can help us overcome them. Everyone has their own combination of things that get in the way of self-care. Some examples might be:

- family and societal messages; for example, that our worth is determined by what we 'do' and 'achieve' or that offering ourselves care is self-indulgent

- busyness or 'doing' offers a convenient distraction from difficult feelings that arise when we pause and quieten

- notions of what it is to be a 'good' and 'helpful' person, which might lead to us prioritizing others' needs over our own.

Self-care is not a selfish act but one of great generosity. In tending to our own needs, we are best placed to support others and avoid burn out. We might think of the flight attendant's instructions that, in the case of an emergency, we should place the oxygen mask on ourselves before tending to others. In modelling self-care, we offer permission for others to follow suit. On many occasions, when I've overcome my inner resistance to saying 'no' or set aside feelings of guilt to carve out space for myself, others have commented that my doing so offered them a valuable reminder to do the same for themselves.

Self-care is something to be patiently nudged towards rather than perfected. We might recognize its value through practising or remember it through noticing the detrimental impact of neglecting it. In either case, slowly but surely over time (which can be years!), our self-care muscle can grow stronger and become easier to implement, as I've found myself.

REFLECTIONS

- What do you feel are your barriers to self-care?

- How might you challenge them?

Chapter 6

HOLDING SPACE FOR OURSELVES

While it's important that much of our awareness rests on our students when teaching, it's equally important that some rests back on ourselves, noticing how *we* are feeling, *our* posture, *our* breathing, opening to the thoughts and feelings that move through *us* while teaching. Doing so supports both ourselves and our students.

Many of us drawn to working in caring professions might be considered 'empaths', being sensitive to and impacted by the feelings of others. As we saw in Section 1, empathy is an essential element in compassion, enabling to sense when others are suffering and being drawn to help alleviate it. But when empathy is not matched with compassion (both for us and others) it can lead to exhaustion. There are some who argue that the commonly termed 'compassion fatigue' that contributes to burn out could more accurately be thought of as 'empathy fatigue', and this really resonates with me.

Our nervous system is sensitive to and impacted by those around us. Being in the company of someone who is sad can leave us feeling flat, whereas we might find ourselves feeling relaxed in the presence of someone calm. This is sometimes known as 'emotional contagion'.

When we are depleted, we tend to be more 'emotionally contagious', the feelings of others seeping more deeply within us. It is like the boundaries between ourselves and others are more permeable. When we are more rested and resourced, they are less porous. When our own self-care has been neglected, we are more prone to absorbing what is being expressed or released by students and subsequently more tired by teaching. When more resourced and resilient, our boundaries feel stronger. We are still able to empathize but there feels sufficient space to compassionately 'hold' the other, without getting submerged in or taking on their experiences.

An image that comes to mind is someone having trouble in turbulent waters. We can support both ourselves and the person in difficulty best when we are safely grounded on the shore throwing a life belt out to them, not when floundering in the choppy water with them. Remaining connected to ourselves when teaching enables us to maintain a grounded, compassionate presence from which we can best support ourselves and our students.

Our capacity for *self*-awareness enables us to sense whether we are on the shore or being pulled into the waters. In remaining attentive to our posture, our breath, the thoughts and feelings moving through us, we can regularly regulate ourselves back to a place of steadiness when needed.

At times, our students will be in the foreground of our awareness while we hold ourselves in a softer focus; at others, it will be the reverse, like a gentle dance that shifts as it needs to. On many occasions when I've held space for someone experiencing strong emotions, I've felt this dance play out within me, enabling my heart to remain open and attentive to both myself and my students.

PRACTICE: MINI CHECK-INS

Offering ourselves a Mini Check-In needn't take long, but offers us a moment to connect with and tend to ourselves, if needed. Take a moment to become aware of:

- *Your posture*: How might you adapt it if needed to feel grounded and steady? Tune into your contact points with the ground and allow them to feel rooted and steady. Feel your spine lengthening from your base, becoming upright, open and at ease.

- *Your body*: Notice places of tension that might soften. For me, it is often the jaw, the shoulders or the belly.

- *Your gaze*: Could it soften, opening to what is before you with soft eyes and a kind heart?

- *Your thoughts and feelings*: If it's helpful, silently name what is moving through you (e.g., 'tension', 'tiredness', 'uncertainty', 'doubt'), acknowledging it without getting caught up in the stories that come with it.

- *Your breathing*: Sense the natural flow of your breath at the belly, if needed imagine being soothed by the inhale and steadied by the exhale.

Practising pausing

For many of us, pausing is something we need to consciously practise. Tendencies towards doing, doing, doing can lead to spaces feeling like things that need 'filling'. But pauses are essential in tuning into how *we* are feeling. As Tara Brach reminds us: 'Until we stop our mental busyness, stop our endless activities, we have no way of knowing our actual experience.'[1]

Pauses needn't be long to be impactful. Small pockets found in a few breaths or minutes can offer precious space to gather ourselves, gain perspective and access greater steadiness. Longer periods, between clients, classes or by way of retreats or holidays, ensure that our work is sustainable.

PRACTICE: STOP

A short, simple practice that encourages us to pause is STOP. This simple acronym reminds us of the power of stopping, stepping out of auto-pilot and opening mindfully to the moment we are in. Take a moment to:

Stop what you are doing and pause.

Take a breath – feel the sensations of your breathing.

> Observe whatever is moving through your experience – the sounds you hear, sensations within your body, thoughts and feelings. Hold them spaciously.
>
> Proceed with what you were doing, but mindfully and compassionately.
>
> It can be surprising how this short moment to pause can impact how we proceed.

Short practices like this can be particularly helpful in moments when we are triggered or overwhelmed, shifting us from our sympathetic nervous system (fight/flight mode) towards our parasympathetic nervous system (sometimes, referred to as tend and befriend mode) where we have access to our calmer, more rational mind and intuitive wisdom.

While we may feel self-conscious offering ourselves a moment to pause *mid*-teaching, doing so can benefit both ourselves and our students. We might offer them a pose in which their gaze rests away from us (Child's Pose can be helpful) and guide them to tune inwards towards their experience. Even offering this for a few breaths will be valuable to their practice while offering ourselves a moment to tend to ourselves.

REFLECTIONS

- How would you define your own relationship to pausing?

- Take a moment to take the STOP practice. What do you notice?

Preparing ourselves for teaching

Take a moment to consider how you prepare and care for yourself before teaching. Do you have any simple, small rituals that support you? Here are some suggestions that may be helpful.

- Arrive to a teaching space early. Give yourself time to land and tend to yourself before students arrive. This can include simple things like going to the toilet or having a drink available to stay hydrated. This may seem obvious but can get missed when sidelined by students arriving. In fact, toilets are often undervalued as spaces where we can take a moment to ourselves, to pause and check in, without anyone questioning it. I carry a calming essential oil roller around with me and find rubbing it on my temples and wrists before teaching is a simple gesture that reminds me that my own needs in this space are important too (as well as being soothed by the smell). When appropriate, lighting candles might feel a marker of switching modes and connecting to light in service of both yourself and your students. A teacher on one of my trainings reflected that by reframing this time before teaching as personal time, she was offering herself (rather than studio time she wasn't being paid for) really helped her in prioritizing and benefiting from it.

- Take a moment to check in with how you are feeling. This allows whatever you bring with you to teaching to feel seen and held, rather than being an unconscious force lurking beneath the surface. While we may not have time to sit in meditation, we can offer this to ourselves in other ways, while calmly walking through the space as we set up, or by taking the STOP practice or the Mini Check-In as students settle at the start.

- Connect to your intention for teaching. Connecting to our heartfelt intention for teaching can help us to feel inspiration and trust in what we are sharing (see Chapter 10).

REFLECTION

– How do you look after your own needs before teaching?

Balancing giving and receiving

In extended moments of quietness and stillness (e.g., when holding space for students in *Śavāsana* or restorative yoga), you might try this simple practice. On days when we feel depleted or disconnected it can remind us of the power and importance of both giving *and receiving* care and kindness.

I found this practice particularly helpful when teaching a lot online. I sometimes missed the energy created by being in the same space as my students. This practice helped my heart to stay open and connected to myself and those I was teaching, feeling nourished by the process (even though students appeared in small boxes on the screen).

PRACTICE: GIVING AND RECEIVING

- Sense into your posture and allow it to feel steady, open, alert but relaxed. Keep your eyes open with a soft gaze on those you are teaching.

- Take your attention to your chest/heart space, sense how your posture supports it in being open and spacious.

- Connect to a sense of common humanity, sensing how both we and our students experience joys and challenges.

- Tune into your breathing and the qualities it offers of both receiving and releasing.

- As you inhale, let your heartfelt attention rest on yourself, imagine drawing in nourishment, care and kindness for yourself.

- As you exhale, let your heartfelt attention rest on your students, imagine sending nourishment, care and kindness towards them and whatever they may be going through.

Clearing and closing after teaching

I often feel energized while teaching, but it is after that I notice the energy expended. If we are teaching numerous classes per week, this can be accumulatively tiring, particularly if we are running from one thing to the next without acknowledging and 'clearing' what we may be unconsciously absorbing while teaching.

Again, I find that small rituals are helpful in prioritizing care for myself after teaching. Some suggestions are to:

- Wash your hands or splash your face with cold water (a favourite of mine when teaching online is to spray my face with a hydrating mist), imagine anything you don't need to carry with you after the class being cleansed away.

- Take a moment in nature to feel held and resourced by forces bigger than yourself.

- Take a gentle shake out (of either the arms or whole body), a sigh and imagine sending anything that needs clearing to an open window or the earth.

- Burn a sage smudge stick (known for its energetic cleansing effects) within the space or around yourself.

REFLECTION

- What do you do to care for yourself after teaching?

Meeting ourselves on difficult days

As teachers we are not saintly figures but human beings. There will be days when we arrive to teach feeling resourced, inspired and resilient. There will be others when we feel distracted, disconnected and destabilized by things we are navigating in our personal or professional lives.

As yoga teachers, we can often be exceptionally hard on ourselves on difficult days, firing second arrows of 'I'm a yoga teacher, I shouldn't feel like this', 'I'm a fraud', 'Who am I to be standing up here teaching?'. On such days, we might feel vulnerable and exposed or pressured to put on a face that we're not feeling inside. This can feel tiring.

On such days, we might consider ways of meeting ourselves more tenderly. Some suggestions when teaching are to:

- Create extra space to tend to ourselves before and around our teaching.

- Give ourselves permission to pull back a little from 'giving', trusting that offering 70% of what we normally would is OK and enables us to care for ourselves while caring for those before us.

- Stay closer to your own mat than you might normally do if this helps you to feel steady and resourced.

- Keep guidance simple and spacious, trusting in the power of the practices.

- Allow your words to be heard as much by yourself as those before you, remembering that we are all on this path of practising not perfecting.

It can be helpful to reframe such days, appreciating that rather than making us 'bad' teachers, they can make us more empathic and compassionate ones. I know for myself that the teachers that most resonate with me are those who talk about the reality of being human rather than claiming to have superseded life's difficulties. The more we practise opening our hearts towards ourselves on such days, the more our hearts open to those before us, appreciating that everyone has vulnerabilities that lie beneath the surface.

REFLECTIONS

- What narratives do you bring to your teaching on difficult days?
- How can you be kind to yourself on such days?

Tapping into sources of steadiness

Just as life has ups and downs, so does teaching. There may be days when classes are full of peaceful looking students and we feel clear that we *love* teaching. Other days, when sessions are quiet or we interpret a student's gaze as dissatisfaction, our confidence flounders. How can we support ourselves in finding steadiness amid these natural fluctuations, seeing them clearly, meeting them calmly and holding them kindly?

The Buddha talked of navigating life amidst what he termed the Eight Worldly Winds[2]

Pleasure and pain,

gain and loss,

praise and blame,

fame and disrepute.

Finding ways to tap into sources of steadiness can help us cultivate equanimity when the force of these winds is blustery. Doing so can feel like dropping anchor, rooting into something solid and steady to embody these qualities within ourselves.

Here, we will explore a couple of meditations using imagery to support us in tapping into qualities of steadiness.

PRACTICE: MOUNTAIN MEDITATION[3]

Although not a formal mindfulness meditation (as it asks us to visualize a scene rather than tune into our present moment experience), the Mountain Mediation can be useful for connecting to a quality of equanimity.

It can help us to appreciate the transient nature of life, that things come and go, there is pleasure and pain but ultimately there is always change. Through our mindfulness practice and this Mountain Meditation we can learn to witness this change from a steadier place.

- Take a moment to find a comfortable seat that enables you to feel steadily connected to the ground (see Chapter 20 for suggested seated meditation postures).

- Draw your attention to the points of contact between yourself and the earth. Tune into the sensations that you feel here. Sense yourself dropping into the firm support of the ground.

- Now, bring to mind an image of a mountain (either one from memory or one imagined). Notice its inherent qualities, its solid base, its sloping sides, how its peak reaches towards the sky.

- Bring to your mind's eye what moves across and around its surface (streams, grass, trees, snow, animals, people). Sense the shifts experienced by the mountain amid changing conditions (e.g., from day to night, varying weathers and seasons).

- Sense how the mountain is steady, grounded and unwavering in its stillness regardless of external conditions.

- Now imagine embodying the qualities of the mountain within yourself – your seat like the steady foundation of the mountain, your head like its peak, your shoulders and arms like its sloping sides.

- Observe what moves through your experience, opening to the sensations in the body, the thoughts and emotions in the heart/mind. Imagine holding them as the mountain does, being a steady, calm witness to the changing weather of our own inner and outer lives.

PRACTICE: STANDING TALL LIKE A GREAT TREE

This meditation is similar to the Mountain Meditation but can offer us a feeling of rooting into steadiness when we are standing.

- Come to a standing posture with your feet slightly apart so that you feel steady and grounded. Tune into the connection of your feet against the ground and the sensations you experience here.

- Bring to mind the image of a great tree, standing firm and tall, branches cast wide.

- Imagine embodying the qualities of the tree within yourself.

- Imagine roots extending from your feet deep into the earth. Feel how the roots and the earth are supporting you.

- Become aware of your posture. Imagine your lower body (from the diaphragm down to your feet) being like the trunk of the tree, strong and steady. You might rest your attention here for a moment, feeling your breath in the abdomen.

- Allow your spine to lengthen, tall and dignified, as if reaching for the sunlight.

- As you feel into your upper body, see where you might soften (e.g., the face, shoulders, arms, heart) allowing for greater ease. Imagine the branches of the tree soft and adaptable to shifts in the weather and seasons.

- Imagine that, like a tree, you have sufficient firmness in your foundation and flexibility in your adaptability that life's winds can move through you without being uprooted or destabilized.

Both the mountain and tree meditations could be taken as a stand-alone practice over a number of minutes, or the images could be brought to mind in short moments when you are in need of tapping into sources of steadiness (whether seated or standing) in daily life or when teaching.

Mindful Walking

At times when stillness is neither accessible nor appropriate, Mindful Walking offers a simple practice to tap into a quality of grounding. It can either be taken as a formal meditation practice (which I highly recommend trying for 10–20 minutes) or an informal practice when walking in daily life.

PRACTICE: MINDFUL WALKING (FORMAL PRACTICE)

This practice could be taken inside or outside. I prefer to take this either in socks or bare feet to allow greater sensitivity in feeling the sensations of my feet against the ground.

- Find a space where you can create a clear path to either walk back and forth or in a circular direction for at least a few metres.

- Before starting, take a moment to pause and drop your attention downwards towards your feet. Sense where they connect with and lift from the earth. Become aware of sensations (pressure, temperature, tingling or numbness, whether toes bunch or spread). Notice if one foot takes more weight than the other. Become curious.

- As you begin to walk, do so as if in slow motion. Feel as one foot slowly lifts from the earth and the weight shifts to the other foot. Sense as the heel makes contact with the ground before weight shifts to the ball of the foot. Now feel the other heel lift and repeat as you walk, bringing in attitudes of mindful awareness.

- If you are walking back and forth, pause for a moment at the 'end' of the path to tune into your experience, before turning and walking back.

- As you continue to walk, you can both broaden and narrow your focus; at times, opening to the whole body, at others, staying with the sensations of the feet, or noticing the movement of the arms, the flow of the breath.

- Notice how it feels to not be striving to *get* somewhere but to simply be with the sensations of walking. The mind may be focussed or distracted, calm or frustrated. Does your pace or movement change when the mind wanders?

PRACTICE: MINDFUL WALKING (INFORMAL PRACTICE)

When taking Mindful Walking into everyday life, we needn't walk as slowly (passersby may think us strange!) but we can still allow our focus to shift to our connection to the earth as we do.

I find this often makes me aware of tendencies towards rushing and reminds me to slow down, to shift out of my head and into my body, to come back to my breathing and feel more grounded and steadier. It helps me remember to open to my senses, becoming present to the environment I'm walking through rather than being lost in thought. I use this often, both when I'm on my way to teaching and while moving through a teaching space.

REFLECTION

- What tools help you feel grounded, calm and present when teaching?

Chapter 7

MEETING AND MANAGING OUR INNER CRITIC

While some of life's difficulties are caused by external conditions, many are created (or aggravated) by the narratives in our heads. You've probably heard the term the 'inner critic' and most likely felt its presence. It's the berating, internal voice that rears its head to say, 'You're *such* an idiot!', '*Who* do you *think* you are!?' or 'I told you, you couldn't do it!'. It is a common companion that many of us carry with us through life, often mistakenly believing its voice to be true.

We might dream of a day (when we have done 'sufficient' training or proved our success) when our inner critic will vanish, but the truth is that, if we choose to grow, explore and move beyond our comfort zone, it will likely come along for the ride.

Let's take a moment to explore it.

REFLECTIVE PRACTICE

Take a moment to look at the following qualities (you might notice how your body responds to the different words):

supporting us with our weaknesses   harsh/critical

only noticing our weaknesses   ignoring our strengths

judgemental   considerate

fair minded   supportive

berating   unhelpful

encouraging   noticing our strengths

friendly/approachable   unfriendly

- First, circle those that you would find helpful in a mentor or employer, qualities that would help you to feel motivated, valued and performing at your best.

- Now, underline those that you seek in friends, qualities that would help you feel calm, happy and supported.

- Finally, ask yourself which most closely match how you talk to yourself in your head.

I do this exercise regularly with young people I work with through a charity supporting them into employment. In asking them which qualities they value in their Job Coaches, there is generally unanimous agreement that qualities of friendliness, considerateness, encouragement, support with weaknesses, noticing strengths, etc., are what bring out the best in them. When the final question is revealed, eyes roll and heads shake as they realize how much this contrasts with how they are with themselves.

I've met many people who believe that without this critical inner narrative they wouldn't get anything done or strive to be their best. However, a vast body of research shows that rather than our inner critic helping us, it hinders us, feeding patterns of stress, anxiety and depression, fearing, and feeling defined by, failure rather than taking healthy risks from which we learn and grow. Cultivating a more compassionate relationship with ourselves promotes greater creativity, growth (being able to learn from mistakes rather than feeling defined by them), calm, clear thinking (as we move from the sympathetic to the parasympathetic nervous system), productivity and resilience.

Meeting ourselves with kindness doesn't mean we don't hold ourselves accountable for our actions or mistakes, but rather that we can see and respond to them skilfully, rather than getting stuck in loops of self-blame or criticism. As Sharon Salzberg writes in her book, *Real Love*:

> Real love allows for failure and suffering. All of us have made mistakes and some of those mistakes were consequential, but you can find a way to relate to them with kindness. No matter what troubles have befallen you or what difficulties you have caused yourself or to others, with love for yourself you can change, grow, make amends and learn. Real love is not about letting ourselves off the hook. Real love does not encourage you to ignore your problems or deny your mistakes and imperfections. You see them clearly and still opt for love.[1]

It can be helpful to remind ourselves that our inner critic comes from a fearful part of our brain intent on keeping us safe. While its narrative may not be nice to live with, its intention is one of protection. Its energy may feel angry and hurtful but it is often simply fearful. It would rather keep us safe and small than go into the unknown.

While mindfulness and compassion may not banish our inner critic, they do offer us greater choice in how we manage it. Mindfulness helps us notice when it dominates, enabling us to step back and consider its viewpoint from a more fair-minded, less fearful perspective, whether its messages are or aren't valid.

In *True Refuge*, Tara Brach suggests using the phrase 'real but not true'[2] when we are caught in unhelpful patterns of thinking. This small phrase helps us to acknowledge that while something may *feel* very real, it doesn't mean it is true. Such phrases may help us to perceive our inner critic as a temporary force moving through us, rather than feeling like a truth deep within us.

While our inner critic offers one perspective, self-compassion reminds us to access other, more supportive ones. On days when our inner critic is dominating the show, we might imagine tucking it up in a restorative pose in the next room so that it can calm down and take a much-needed break!

REFLECTIONS

- When does your inner critic tend to show up? Maybe when you're tired, stressed or doing something for the first time?

- What kind of manner does it have (e.g., angry, dismissive, belittling, harsh, hostile)?

- What kind of words or phrases does it fire at you?

- If you were to personify it, how would it look and what name would you give it? You might choose to bring in some humour here.

Cultivating compassionate inner companions

While it might not be possible (or always helpful) to banish our inner critic, we can choose to cultivate more compassionate inner companions to accompany, soothe and settle it. Paul Gilbert describes this aspect of ourselves as our 'compassionate self'.[3] We might think of having a boardroom in our brain. While our inner critic can be a rather loud, boisterous participant, can we learn to bring some more rational, caring members to the table to counterbalance it? For me, this has been one of the most transformative tools in my self-care toolbox.

This reminds me of the Native American legend in which a grandfather is talking with his grandson to explain that there are two wolves inside of us which are always at battle. One is a good wolf which represents things like kindness, bravery, love and connection. The other is a lone wolf, which represents things like greed, hatred and fear. The grandson considers this and asks, 'Grandfather, which one wins?', to which the grandfather replies, 'The one you feed'.

Many of us spend years believing and feeding our inner critic's narratives. Cultivating new, more compassionate inner companions may feel strange or clunky initially, but with regular practice, they become more familiar and comfortable visitors. As with anything new, it can be helpful to take things slowly and meet ourselves patiently. We might think of lifting weights at the gym – we would build up progressively, not reach for 50kg weights on our first visit. Similarly, we can gently nudge our way forward with meeting ourselves more kindly.

Finding a kinder inner narrative can take a little exploring. It may be helpful initially to bring to mind a caring friend or loved one and imagine them talking to you. What words would they say? What would their tone of voice be like? In what ways would they express care and kindness? You might consider terms of affection that they would call you (e.g., 'my love', 'honey', 'sweetheart', 'my dear' or 'mate') and use this towards yourself. Initially, it can feel a bit silly, but in my own experience, it becomes a more familiar, natural companion over time.

PRACTICE: SELF-COMPASSION BREAK[4]

In moments when we recognize that we are suffering, we can remember to pause and direct compassion towards ourselves.

Kristin Neff's 'Self-Compassion Break' is a beautiful practice for such moments. It draws on the three core components of self-compassion (mindfulness, self-kindness and common humanity).

- Bring to mind a situation that is causing you some difficulty. (Note: Avoid choosing something that is likely to feel traumatic or overwhelming; start with something that feels manageable).

- As you feel into this scenario, bring a mindful attention to your experience. Rather than pulling away, gently explore it. What do you notice happening in your body, what thoughts and feelings arise? What are you believing?

- Tenderly offer yourself some words to acknowledge what you are feeling, such as, 'I'm finding this difficult', 'this feels hard just now' or 'this is a moment of suffering'.

- Now, connect to your sense of common humanity, acknowledging how normal and understandable it is to feel this way. You are not alone. Difficult times are a part of everyone's life.

- Tenderly offer yourself some words that acknowledge this, such as 'it's really normal to feel like this', 'you're not alone, others feel like this too sometimes'.

- Now sense how you might bring some kindness towards yourself in this moment. This might take the form of caring touch, placing one or both hands over your chest or gently stroking your hand or head, allowing yourself to feel and receive warmth and tenderness.

- Tenderly offer yourself some words of care and support, such as, 'I'm here for you' or 'may I be kind to myself in this moment'. If this feels difficult bring a dear friend to mind and imagine what they might say to you in this moment or what caring action they would suggest (perhaps to take a break, get some fresh air or make a cup of tea). See if you can offer this to yourself.

Take a moment to reflect on anything you notice while you did this.

This is a practice that we might sit with for a few minutes when we have time and space, or else combine it into three short phrases when in the midst of everyday life (e.g., 'this feels difficult just now', 'it's normal to feel like this', 'may I be kind to myself in this moment').

We might sense how our critical inner narrative tends to feed our threat response (whether fight, flight or freeze), as if guarding ourselves against the threat of not being good enough, or not belonging. However, our more compassionate self stimulates the ventral vagal aspect of the parasympathetic nervous system[5] where we feel safety, calmness and connection (sometimes referred to as 'tend and befriend' mode). I know for myself I often sense my body softening, my breath deepening and my mind calming when taking this practice. While it doesn't make our pain and difficulties go away, it offers us a calmer, kinder container in which to hold them, it enables us to soothe ourselves when in the midst of them, and, therefore, reduces additional suffering.

Culling comparisons

Inner critics are easily fed on comparisons. In our age of social media, where selective and often heavily edited versions of people's lives display perpetual happiness, success and abundance, our sense of self-worth is often gauged against unrealistic perceptions of others. Without careful management, we can be drawn into false narratives that leave us feeling isolated and falling short and then driven to compete and compensate.

Creating caring connections which allow us to see and be seen in an authentic capacity can help to minimize this. Certainly, for me, managing my relationship to social media is high up there in practising self-care. Another is ensuring that I get oxytocin hits by connecting with teachers in real life (whether on the phone, online or in person). Such interactions can make us feel held within a caring community rather than fuelling feelings of comparison and competition.

Celebrating our successes

As we have seen in Section 1, our brain's inherent negativity bias steers our awareness towards noticing the negative rather than the positive. Without careful attention, this can skew our perception of ourselves and our abilities.

Taking time to consciously celebrate our successes and soak up what is good within our teaching offers us a more balanced and accurate perspective, enabling us to acknowledge our strengths and competencies and increase our sense of confidence and resilience.

Let's explore some ways you might do this.

PRACTICE: CELEBRATE OUR SUCCESSES

- *Appraising ourselves:* If working in a freelance capacity we don't receive appraisals from employers but we can create time and space (whether monthly or annually) to offer this to ourselves. Doing so allows us to step back from the detail of the to-do list and see the bigger picture, to celebrate our strengths and successes, to acknowledge what lights us up and what we have brought into being. This can be done during a moment alone with a cup of tea and a note pad or gathering with fellow teachers to consider it collectively.

- *Savouring the good:* As we have seen in Section 1, positive experiences slip from our brains like Teflon unless we consciously choose to pay attention to them. (Again, in his practice 'Internalizing the Positive', Rick Hanson suggests for 5–20 seconds.)[6]

  When you receive positive feedback or feel uplifted by the impact of your work, take a moment to pause and really let it soak in, bringing the event back to mind, imagining the scene, remembering the words that were said and how you felt inside, allowing the good feelings to fully embed.

- *Saving the good:* Create space to store positive feedback (e.g., nice cards, emails or words of thanks relating to your teaching). I have both a physical box and an email folder called 'Nice emails', which is lovely to dip into on days when self-doubt creeps in.

REFLECTIONS

Take a moment to:

- write down three things you do well

- celebrate three recent successes in your teaching

- bring to mind some positive feedback from someone who you've taught and take a moment to soak it in.

Chapter 8

HEALTHY BOUNDARIES

In Section 3, we will explore how healthy boundaries support our students in feeling seen, safe and held when practising. Here, let's consider how they can support us as teachers.

While the word 'boundaries' can conjure up images of harsh, defensive walls that divide one another, I love Prentis Hemphill's description: 'Boundaries are the distance at which I can love you and me simultaneously'.[1] I find this helpful, seeing boundaries as something that enables both parties to be respected and cared for while they interact (rather than barriers to keep them apart).

Yoga can sometimes be viewed as a caring profession and, as such, teachers should be unlimited in their offering. This may lead some to question how we charge for our services or cancellation fees. While we may offer flexibility in varying circumstances, having clearly defined policies relating to this can enable us to feel more comfortable and confident in acknowledging and stating our worth and needs.

For some, it can feel rare to be seen and held in a compassionate setting. It is understandable that some students may wish for more of our attention than we have, either in terms of time, energy or what is appropriate, given the nature of our role. As teachers, we serve our students best through being caring, approachable *and* professional, without falling into a friendship role. Being clear on how and when we are available to our students outside of the class context can be helpful, perhaps stating that we have 'a few minutes' after teaching for questions, but being clear when what is requested is inappropriate or requires personal tuition.

Similarly, some may feel (or we may feel ourselves) that being a compassionate person involves *always* being there for others. Many of us have a people-pleasing tendency that frequently leads us to saying 'yes' far more than we have either time or energy for. Learning to say 'no' (and not feel guilty for it!) when needed has been one of the most significant acts of self-compassion that I now practise. Often, I feel the 'yes' rising to the surface and remember to pause, then say something like: 'That sounds really interesting, let me get back to you about that'. Only when I've had time to truly consider if I have the interest and capacity for it do I respond. A helpful question here is: 'What value is our yes, if we never say no?'

REFLECTION

- In what ways do you create boundaries to support your well-being?

Sustainable scheduling

Our experiences of teaching will understandably vary: full or part-time, urban or more rural setting, the only teacher in the area or one of many. While such factors inevitably influence our opportunities and choices, it can be helpful to step back and consider how our schedule is supporting our sustainability.

At times, particularly when new to teaching and eager to gain experience, it may be necessary to say yes to opportunities that are less than ideal (e.g., taking on classes further afield or at times that aren't best fitting). While this might be sustainable for a short period, we may need to regularly assess whether our own wellbeing is being sacrificed in doing so.

PRACTICE: REVIEWING YOUR SCHEDULE

- How many classes feel appropriate to teach? While 10–15 classes may not sound a lot, once travel, planning and admin time are added, it is more realistically a 35-hour week.

- Do you intentionally create sufficient spaces between classes or clients to offer yourself moments to both 'land' and 'clear' before and after sessions?

- Consider the natural rhythms that you are influenced by. For example:

  - Are you an early bird or a night owl (or somewhere in-between)?

  - Is there a time of day when your energy naturally dips? Can you intentionally use this as a time to offer yourself conscious rest?

  - How are you affected by hormonal or seasonal cycles and can you be considerate to this?

- If teaching across vast distances, do your fees adequately reflect your travel time? Can your schedule be shaped so that you offer work in particular locations over extended periods to reduce distances travelled?

- Do you prioritize days off? Earning a sustainable income from teaching can be challenging. Trying to keep at least one full day a week personal and precious – no classes, no cover, no emails – is not only compassionate, it is essential for our physical, mental and emotional health. That's why weekends developed!

- When you consider your teaching schedule, what depletes your energy? Perhaps it is a particular class or an activity. Personally, I find city transport over-stimulating and screen time depleting. Too much online teaching might drain us and need to be balanced with more face-to-face teaching.

- Consider what nourishes and sustains you. This might relate to *what* you are teaching. My teaching style has changed over the years; this is natural as we move through life – we age, priorities and interests change. Classes we once loved teaching might now leave us feeling deflated and something needs to change. This can feel scary, particularly if we have built a steady stream of students. Staying attentive to what lights us up and what leaves us depleted allows our teaching to come from a place of authenticity. We can trust that students will find us when we are inspired and energized by our teaching.

Take a moment to consider what nourishes your *ānanda-maya kośa* (see Chapter 1) both within *and* outside of teaching, connecting you to feelings of peace, lightness and joy? Do you consciously schedule this in? Maybe time in nature, time with friends and family, dancing, visiting galleries, cooking, doing DIY, quietly reading. The list is endless. My favourite has become feeding the ducks in my local park.

In identifying what nourishes and drains us, we can consider where changes can be made. Of course, some drainers might simply be a part of life (housework, emails, travel) but we can consider whether we are building in sufficient sustainers to counterbalance them and resource ourselves.

REFLECTION

- How might you change your schedule to make it more sustainable?

Valuing our worth

For some, discussions around yoga and finances can feel uncomfortable, even controversial. Over the years, I've heard people describe financial negotiations as 'unyogic', that our teaching should come from a place of entirely selfless service.

Few of us come to teaching motivated by financial gain. More often, it is a heart-felt desire to share these powerful practices, having felt their benefit in our own lives. Decisions and discussions around finances aren't about being greedy but rather valuing our worth and creating conditions for sustainability.

When considering our fees we need to consider not only our time directly teaching but our time in planning, travelling, marketing, answering emails, not to mention the costs of insurance, belonging to professional bodies, setting aside money for professional development. Ensuring that we can afford to take time off when sick or in need of a break (as well as save for a pension) is self-compassion in action.

We pay professional rates for our training; it is fair to ask for an income that reflects our level of training, experience, time and expenses. Otherwise, we run the very real risk of teaching being restricted to the privileged few who don't need an income.

REFLECTIONS

- What are your thoughts on self-care in relation to finances?

- Are there any changes you might make?

Chapter 9

SEEKING SUPPORT

Mindfulness and compassion can help us to foresee and minimize some of the difficulties we experience in life. However, difficult days will inevitably arise. Again, while self-compassion enables us to be a part of our own support network, we shouldn't be its sole member. On days when we can't see our own light or find stability, the kindest thing we can do for ourselves is to reach out for support externally.

As well as holding space for others, we need space held for ourselves; spaces where we can show up honestly, share openly and be met non-judgementally. At times it can be helpful to do this with our peers, at other times with a mentor or supervisor who is a little further travelled along the path than us. Whatever their nature, such connections can feel like beacons of light to look out for and move towards on foggy days.

Peer support

Meeting with fellow teachers enables us to feel nourished and supported by connection and community. Many spiritual traditions, including yoga, recognize the importance of *saṅgha*, gathering with like-minded people on a similar path.

Connecting with our peers offers space to share ideas, remain inspired, to laugh and offload. It can offer external eyes to remind us of our capabilities as well as opportunities to be healthily and respectfully challenged.

I have a group of fellow teachers without whom I don't think I could have found my way through the ups and downs of teaching. Some I intentionally connect with regularly. Doing so provides a regular check in, an opportunity to reflect on what inspires or frustrates us, and a time to celebrate successes, as well as consider what we want to bring into fruition or be held accountable to.

Monthly teachers' gatherings are another option, providing an informal opportunity to make and sustain connections. Working in a freelance profession can feel isolating and peer support can help us feel a part of a supportive collective rather than competitively pitched against one another (particularly if our main source of connection is via social media).

Mentoring and supervision

It often surprises me that mentoring and supervision aren't a requirement for yoga teachers. While we may not be therapists (unless we are trained as such), our work is often therapeutic in nature. As we hold space for others, much can arise (both within ourselves and our students) and mentoring and supervision offer a space for this to be held and explored, for us to learn and grow. There is much to be gained by accessing the support of people more experienced than us, teachers who have travelled a similar path but bring their years of experience with them as they accompany us on ours.

Mentoring can take different forms, either in a group setting or one-to-one. It might include an element of structured guidance and training as well as space to share and receive support. In the group supervision sessions I've attended as a yoga therapist, I've welcomed the opportunity to share ideas and learn from my peers as well as the more experienced therapist facilitating.

I have found working one-to-one with a supervisor over many years so beneficial. In a profession where much can change, this constancy can be invaluable, being witnessed and compassionately held as I both stumble and grow. Supervision sessions provide a safe space for difficult feelings to be aired, space for reflection and challenges to be explored. Sometimes, they allow us to develop competencies in challenging situations, other times they shine a light on existing capabilities when we can't see them.

Ultimately, these relationships create precious spaces where we can feel seen, safe and supported rather than so alone. Such support does come with a financial cost, but from my own experience, it forms an aspect of my support network that I couldn't do without.

REFLECTIONS

- In what ways do you currently access support?

- In what ways do you feel your support network could be strengthened?

SELF-CARE ACTION PLANNING

In Section 3 our focus will shift towards our students. Before doing so, take a moment to consider action points from this section that would support yourself.

- What are the key areas that you feel detrimentally impact your wellbeing and sustainability?

- What are the main changes you would like to create with regards to self-care?

- When considering the *kośas* (see Chapter 1), in what ways do you plan to notice and tend to:

  - your body

  - your vital energy

  - your mental and emotional health

  - your intuitive wisdom

  - nourishing your spirit with qualities of peace and joy?

- What small act of self-care and kindness would you like to build into every day?

MINDFUL, COMPASSIONATE TEACHING

'Instead of measuring success in practicing a Yoga posture by how far we go, we can ask how present we are in each moment. How aware are we of the movement of our breath, the sensations in our body, and the thoughts that pass through us?'

Donna Farhi[1]

Overview

While the nature of our teaching will no doubt vary, offering space for people to practise is precious. For some students, it might be the only time in the week (or month) that they let go of their daily 'doing', where they allow their attention to rest back on themselves.

We might assume that by teaching yoga, we are automatically steering people towards becoming more connected and embodied, better able to manage their monkey minds and meet the world with an open heart. Yet without careful guidance, it is easy to teach (and practise) on auto-pilot, perpetuating unhelpful patterns rather than counterbalancing them. As teachers, part of our role is to notice the patterns of our students.

Maybe they are operating at a fast pace, with high energy, pounding themselves in their practice and struggling with or even skipping *Śavāsana*, or just doing things half-heartedly and flopping into every pose. Our role as a teacher is to help students move out of auto-pilot and guide them towards awareness and balance.

In this section, we will explore ways of bringing the threads of mindfulness and compassion to the foreground of our teaching in service of our students. We will consider it throughout the journey of our teaching from intention setting, marketing, planning, preparing and when directly teaching.

Chapter 10

INTENTIONS, MOTIVATIONS AND MARKETING

Before we consider our time directly 'teaching', let's step back a little and connect to what guides and inspires our teaching, as well as the messages that we convey when marketing our offerings.

Connecting to our heart-felt intention

Take a moment to consider what motivates and inspires your teaching. What is your heart-felt intention? For me, it is about creating safe spaces where:

- people can reconnect to themselves with care and compassion

- busy, dull or scattered minds can begin to focus

- bodies can be inhabited and befriended where hearts can open and nervous systems can balance

- people sense feelings of connection and belonging

- people learn to listen and respond to their inner wisdom

- people feel more equipped to navigate their life's ups and downs and follow a path more connected with their heart.

In moments of doubt, either about the power of these practices or our ability to share them, our intention can remind us of what matters most to us in teaching. On difficult days, it can help to quieten our inner critic, reminding us that our ability to be a good teacher isn't centred around perfectly choreographed sequences nor our ability to wow students with our own practice. It is not about helping people to get better at performing complex poses (although, of course, there is skill in sequencing wisely and many lessons to be learnt along the journey towards them). It reminds us that we are not here to be perfect but to be human. We are not here to have definitive answers nor fix anyone but rather to be a gentle guide. This can create the conditions through which students can explore *their* experience, listen to insights that arise and deepen their capacity to be led by them in their everyday lives.

REFLECTION

Take a moment to reflect on your own heart-felt intention for teaching.

– What motivates, inspires and drives you within your teaching?

Perceptions of 'progress'

'I'm no good at yoga, I can't even touch my toes!'

This familiar phrase offers a strong indication of how many perceive yoga. In a world where our sense of achievement and success is often action-orientated, quantifiable by visual results, it is understandable how people's perceptions of progress often relate to the performance of physical poses rather than shifts in mental or emotional states.

Given the intrinsic link between minds and bodies, our body offers an important role in accessing peace of mind. Progress in our practice, however, is not determined by the shapes we create with it.

Finding clarity on how we ourselves perceive progress shapes our teaching. In placing presence at the heart of our teaching, we convey to students that progress can be found in many forms, such as their increased ability to:

- focus their attention

- return to presence when their mind wanders

- tune into both strong and subtle sensations

- cultivate attitudes of mindful awareness (e.g., patience, non-judging, curiosity)

- listen to and respond to their intuitive wisdom

- meet themselves and others with compassion.

REFLECTIONS

- How do you define progress within a yoga practice?

- How does this colour your teaching?

Messages and marketing

Some years ago while handing out flyers in my local community, I was intrigued if disheartened by varying responses to the word 'yoga'. Young women often happily reached for a flyer, many men scoffed with an embarrassed 'not for me!', some who fell outside of the common social media representation of a yoga practitioner (young, thin, flexible) looked away. This makes me sad. While I appreciate that yoga isn't for everyone, I would love these common perceptions to change.

We have the opportunity to connect and communicate with actual and potential students in many ways beyond our direct teaching. It can be helpful to consider the messages we impart through various channels (e.g., website, flyers, social media and newsletters) about what yoga is, its benefits and our intention for teaching. This can create yoga spaces that feel welcoming to step into as much as be in.

REFLECTIONS

- Do you find yourself influenced by how you think you 'should' present yourself to be perceived as a skilful teacher?

- How do you convey yourself, your intention and your offering with authenticity?

- How do you convey that yoga is more than *āsana*?

- In what ways do you reflect accessibility, inclusivity and diversity within your marketing?

Chapter 11

HOLDING SPACE

As much as our practice offers space to access greater peace and ease, it also provides space to meet our hard edges, our tensions and distractions. Inviting students to tune into and tend to their experience offers the potential for transformation and healing. It also shines a light on places of vulnerability that need to be held safely, sensitively and skilfully.

I remember a conversation with a Portuguese yoga teacher in which she commented that 'holding space' was such a common term amongst yoga teachers, yet there was no direct translation in Portuguese. This opened an interesting discussion about what we mean by it.

Holding space is perhaps one of the most crucial aspects of our teaching. It is about creating a setting that enables those who step into it to feel seen, safe and held. It encompasses the environment that we create and the qualities we model, creating compassionate containers for the events that arise and unfold within it.

I once received an email from a student saying 'I wanted to thank you for the class. You create such a compassionate "holding" and it was good to be back in my body. It's quite rare for me to feel safe enough to really "be" in my body so I just wanted to feedback what a special gift you have.' This capacity for holding space may seem to our students like an inherent gift that we have, but in reality it is a skill we can all develop.

Our capacity for presence lies at the heart of holding space, enabling us to be attentive to ourselves and those before us, enabling students to feel seen and safely held.

In cultivating our capacity for mindful, compassionate presence in our own practice, it naturally flows into our teaching. As our nervous systems calm, we stimulate what Stephen Porges terms our ventral vagal state[1] and, therefore, our social engagement system. This impacts our body language (being more grounded and open), our facial expressions (becoming more warm and friendly) and our tone of voice (becoming softer and more soothing). Together, this results in our unconsciously signalling social cues of calmness, warmth and kindness, which strengthen feelings of connection and safety to those in our presence.

Mindful, compassionate presence

Take a moment to consider how a teacher's quality of presence impacts your own practice. For example:

- How do you feel when you sense a teacher is fully present?

- How do you feel when a teacher seems disconnected or absorbed in their own practice while teaching?

- How do you feel when a teacher is modelling the attitudes of mindfulness (e.g., being open, non-judgemental, patient, compassionate)?

- How do you feel when these qualities are lacking?

Research points to the fact that in therapy, the most significant factor impacting clients' progress is the ability of the therapist to be present. Although as yoga teachers, we're not therapists (unless trained as such), the practice of yoga is therapeutic in nature and I would argue the same concept applies.

Clinical psychologist Dr Shari Geller defines therapeutic presence as:

> bringing one's whole self into the encounter with a client, being completely in the moment…physically, emotionally, cognitively, spiritually and relationally. Presence also involves being grounded in one's self, while receptively taking in the verbal and bodily expression of the client's in the moment experience.[2]

By connecting to our own embodied experience, as well as our students', we remain attentive to messages we empathically receive about how *they* may be feeling, whilst remaining connected to our intuition offering insights into how we might support them. As Geller adds, 'While this inner receptivity involves therapists' openness to the client's multidimensional internal world, it also involves openness and contact with therapists' own bodily experience in order to access the knowledge, professional skill and wisdom embodied within.'[3]

Holding space well requires us to remain present to ourselves, our students and our environment with a deep, listening presence. In this context, 'listening' is about far more than our ears taking in sounds, but includes what our eyes are seeing, our hearts are feeling and our intuition sensing. It is a full, embodied presence.

In doing so, when teaching, we remain curious and attentive to the message students consciously and unconsciously impart. For example:

- *How they hold their bodies:* Do we detect ease or rigidity, steadiness and balance or being excessively open or closed?

- *How they move:* Are they slow and considered, tentative or fast and furious?

- *How present they appear to be:* Do they seem hypervigilant, scattered, distracted, sleepy or calmly attentive?

- *How easily they settle:* Are they comfortable in stillness, falling asleep or fidgeting?

- *How they breathe:* What is its speed, depth, quality? Where does it flow with ease? Where it is restricted?

- *How easily they access or ask for support:* Do they allow themselves comfort, reach for props or resit them?

- *How they describe their experience:* Particularly when working one-to-one, paying attention to how students describe their felt experience can offer us guidance on how to move them towards balance.

We might notice a correlation or disparity between what students report and what we witness. This can offer insights into how connected and aware they are of themselves. I remember working with a young man who was a city trader experiencing digestive issues. On asking how stress played out in his life he responded. 'Oh, I'm not stressed' as his tightly held and fidgeting body suggested the contrary.

Our capacity for presence enables us to meet our students where they are, ensuring that we are teaching people not poses.

Authenticity

When we begin teaching, we might think we need to mimic how our teacher(s) spoke and held space. Or we might adopt a manner fitting of what we think a yoga teacher *should* be rather than speaking from our hearts. It can take a while to find our own style and voice but trusting in it is important. Adopting a 'yoga teacher voice' rather than our natural voice can leave some students unsure of who the teacher really is. This can impact their ability to place trust in them.

We can sense when someone is being authentic. Practising mindfulness and compassion can help with this. It can enable us to connect more deeply with who we are, trust in what rings true to us and teach from that place. Self-compassion reminds us that we don't have to show up as some other, more 'perfect' teacher. Instead, we show up as our authentic selves and that is enough.

As we embody qualities of mindfulness and compassion (in how we hold ourselves, the students and the space), it is palpable that we are walking the walk as much as talking the talk.

Offering a grounded presence

In Section 2, we explored how taking time to ground ourselves benefits ourselves as teachers. Here, let's consider its benefit for our students.

While we can't be responsible for everything that occurs within a teaching space, we can be attentive and calmly responsive towards it. Through our steady, grounded presence, students sense they are held in a safe container. This enables them to draw their attention inward (rather than remain externally vigilant) assured that we are calmly monitoring and managing the environment.

The way that we sit, stand and move within a space can support this. We can practice Mindful Walking (see Chapter 6) *while* teaching, so that we are attentive and intentional about how we move through a space. We may walk more quickly when students' eyes are open in a standing pose, our pace slowing when eyes are cast low, their attention dropping inwards in, say, a forward fold. As students drop into deep rest, we tread ever more slowly and sensitively, our footsteps respectful to the vulnerability that we bear witness to; becoming an almost imperceptible presence that supports rather than disturbs their practice.

Sitting and standing in ways that support us feeling rooted and grounded (see Chapters 6 and 20) supports students in sensing we offer a calm presence that can steadily hold whatever might arise during practice.

Caring connections

Offering a warm welcome goes a long way in helping people feel a sense of belonging. I know for myself how differently I feel as a student when met with a caring presence. It helps me feel valued and acknowledged as a person, rather than lost in a sea of bodies. It helps me feel that whatever arises as I practice will be held in kindness.

A simple smile goes a long way. Where we can, asking people's names and offering our own promotes a sense of shared connection; yes, we may be the teacher, but we are also human beings.

Staying connected to a sense of our common humanity helps us appreciate that, regardless of what we do or don't know about our students, everyone brings with them personal histories, complexities and vulnerabilities that aren't visible, but need to be held sensitively and respectfully.

The Loving Kindness meditation (see Chapter 20) is a beautiful practice to support us in keeping our hearts open to everyone in a teaching space: to ourselves, those we know well, those who we meet for the first time and even those whose behaviour we find challenging. It connects us to the reality that we are all human, doing the best we can and deserving of care and attention.

Enabling autonomy

To feel held safely within a teaching space, students need to know that they have some autonomy over their practice. This doesn't mean bypassing a teacher's instruction or doing something completely different, but rather that their personal choices about what feels right or wrong for them will be respected; that they won't be forced to do something that doesn't feel appropriate nor shamed for adapting as they need to.

Suitable settings

Teaching spaces needn't be serenely beautiful (although it can be a bonus). I have soaked up the benefits of practice in old church halls, beautiful studios and workspace dining halls. But it can be helpful to consider factors that impact students feeling safely contained and able to tune inwards as they practice.

I remember covering a class in a space that was the access route to all other rooms in a multifunctional community centre. Over the course of the session, numerous visitors passed through; one was curious and asked to watch the class; another was in tears wanting to be directed to a member of staff; another was a workman hired for a job in the space. While it's possible to skilfully hold space in such less-than-ideal conditions (remaining grounded, asking students to pause in a restful pose while managing each visitor), it is challenging, and no doubt impacts those practising. Being in spaces that offer a safe, closed container for practice is beneficial. This offers us some agency on who enters and leaves and greater autonomy over the environment we create within it.

When teaching in a gym setting, it's common for spaces to have mirrors. Setting up the space so that students aren't facing them can highlight a shift in intention, that our practice is more about sensing inwards rather than being drawn to our external appearance.

Of course, undesirable distractions and less than ideal conditions can offer valuable lessons in practising equanimity, but it is helpful if these circumstances are the exception rather than the rule.

Clear boundaries

Section 2 explored how healthy boundaries support our sustainability as teachers. Here, we will consider how they can support students in feeling held safely. Key elements could include the following:

- *Reliability:* Something as simple as starting and ending sessions on time can offer a foundation of security and respects that students have lives and commitments outside of our teaching.

- *Professionalism:* Being clear that we are supporting students in a professional rather than personal capacity. Staying within the limits of our training and capabilities and referring students on to other professionals when their needs fall outside of this.

- *Clarity:* Offering clarity on the terms and conditions of our offerings, responsibilities, pricing, refunds, etc.

- *Confidentiality:* Maintaining confidentiality of information shared by students and informing them of any exceptions to this (e.g., sharing information with a mentor or supervisor, or with external agencies if there is concern that they are a risk to themselves or others). Storing students' personal data in accordance with legislation.

- *Enabling self-agency:* Seeking permission when touching or adjusting students as well as offering agency for students to adapt as they need.

While much of this may seem obvious, take a moment to consider how you feel when these qualities are lacking.

REFLECTION

- What feels important to you in relation to 'holding space' for your students?

Chapter 12

THEMING AND SEQUENCING

How we plan and prepare before teaching will differ. Sometimes, we may arrive and either ask or sense what students need, intuitively building a class around it. Some of us find confidence in coming with a clear plan knowing that we can veer from it as required. Some will come from lineages that teach a set sequence.

Theming

Theming a practice around one of the attitudes of mindful awareness (e.g., beginner's mind, patience, presence, letting go, compassion) can be a lovely way to highlight that our focus is as much about qualities of heart/mind as our physical form.

In weaving these attitudes into our teaching, we can drop in points of inquiry to explore where a quality can be found or lacking, offering ways of cultivating it. We can help students to sense the interplay between the different layers of their being (e.g., how impatience may be found in critical thoughts as well as muscles straining and the breath holding). This can help students to see how unhelpful patterns on the mat might play out in their wider lives. In turn, new, more supportive ways of being may begin to spill from the mat into their everyday lives.

Sequencing

Skilful sequencing involves *vinyāsa krama* – the wise ordering of smaller steps that move us safely and steadily towards a particular point. It can be helpful to consider that this is as much about skilfully guiding minds and hearts as muscles and bones. After all, 'challenging' can mean more than physically demanding. For many, equally (if not more!) challenging than a headstand is being still without agitation, returning to presence when the mind is wandering, or practising self-compassion when uncomfortable feelings surface. In this context, we might consider how our teaching is moving students not just towards a 'peak' pose, but towards qualities of comfort, calmness and focused awareness in *Śavāsana* and meditation.

Offering time at the very start for students to pause, 'land' and meet themselves with a mindful, compassionate presence highlights that this lies at the heart of practice. Doing so offers space to acknowledge their starting point, what is needing care or attention and what their intention is for practising. It helps students sense the importance in simply noticing their experience, without always seeking a particular outcome.

The journey of self-exploration can be a bumpy one in which we meet the familiar and unexplored, the pleasing and unpleasant. For this reason, I like to start with guiding students to notice sources of steadiness, such as the connection of the body against the ground, the flow of the breath, sensing these as steady reference points that can be returned to if needed throughout the practice.

When sequencing *āsana* practices, layering from the simpler to more complex (without a notion of hierarchy) enables students to explore options, progressively pausing at or repeating the one that meets their needs. We can support this by offering variations that hold the same function and similar form (e.g., opening the front body) but with varying levels of intensity. For example, we might build progressively towards Bow Pose by beginning with Half Locust, then Full Locust, before offering Bow Pose as an option to those who find it accessible. Students can then assess which variation best meets their needs that day and stay with it.

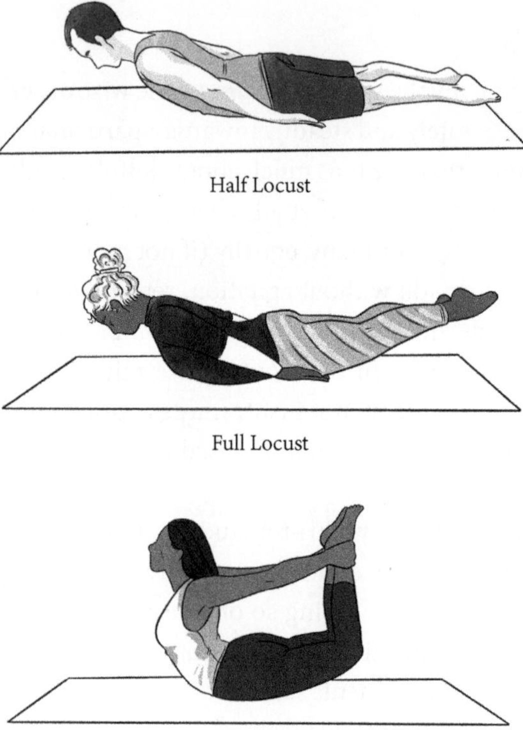

Half Locust

Full Locust

Bow Pose

Doing so supports students in remaining engaged in their practice, sensing the validity of meeting their personal needs rather than only being offered to 'sit out' a pose if it isn't suitable for them. It enables rest to be reframed as something to take when we need or desire it, rather than something that signals we are 'failing' or unable to 'keep up'.

Similarly, when teaching *prāṇāyāma* we can begin with that which is most accessible (e.g., lengthening, smoothing and steadying the breath) before progressively exploring other aspects (e.g., breath ratios and retentions) if appropriate and accessible.

We can layer within our teaching options that encourage students to listen and respond to their unique needs. For example, at times, we might offer a choice between:

- movement or stillness (e.g., flowing between poses or pausing in Child's Pose or Downward Dog)

- stability or challenge (e.g., enjoying both feet feeling firmly rooted or moving into a standing balance)

- softening over support or seeking an active stretch (e.g., Child's Pose with or without a bolster).

Doing so means that in a group setting students can make choices not based on what they 'can' do, but rather on what brings them towards balance in that moment.

Practising slowly and steadily deepens students' capacity to inhabit and listen to their bodies. Doing so stimulates the parasympathetic nervous system (promoting feelings of calm), making stillness more accessible. Incorporating pockets of stillness throughout the practice can prepare students for more extended periods that follow. In this way, our sequencing intentionally guides students towards greater awareness and ease in the stillness of *Śavāsana* and meditation.

Chapter 13

LANGUAGE USE

The words we use matter. It can be helpful, therefore, to consider language use, noticing default phrases we use, habits we fall into and the underlying messages that students unconsciously absorb when practicing.

As we explore language, I want to stress the importance of offering sufficient space and silence *around* our guidance. We will explore this in more depth later, but my recommendation is to think of these as suggestions to be lightly and selectively scattered, allowing sufficient room in the soil that they land on for them to take root, rather than students feeling overwhelmed or zoning out from a dense, overgrown forest of instructions. There have been times when a teacher's guidance has been so incessant that it felt like a background hum I no longer tuned into. On other occasions, a selective phrase would be dropped in such a way that it felt like it sank into my whole being.

At times in this section, suggested phrases are offered. These are intended to spark ideas, encouraging you to explore words that feel authentic to you rather than using mine verbatim.

Guiding towards a state of 'being' as much as 'doing'

In teaching, we will naturally offer instructions regarding what students are 'doing', directing them towards 'moving', 'stretching', 'placing', 'engaging', 'lengthening' or 'softening', etc. It is helpful, however, to be equally proficient in language that guides students towards a state of 'being'.

Broadening and varying our terminology can be helpful in retaining students' interest and engagement. Guidance to '*just notice* X, Y, Z' repeated regularly loses its potency. Alternative words include 'sensing', 'observing', 'witnessing', 'exploring', 'feeling into', 'becoming aware of', 'tuning into' or 'opening to'.

Within our language, we can communicate that awareness is something that can be intentionally:

- *Directed:* inviting students to 'gently guide', 'gather', 'draw' or 'rest' their attention towards the back body, or 'open' to the felt sense of their heart.

- *Broadened:* inviting awareness to 'fill the whole body', how it might feel like a 'spacious container' that they are 'held' within, offering that they allow their attention to broaden to 'open to all that it is to be you in this moment'.

- *Narrowed:* suggesting that they might 'refine' or 'narrow' their attention to the sense of the breath at the nostrils, sensing the aliveness felt in the feet.

- *Imbued with certain qualities:* sensing how their awareness might hold a lightness, softness, warmth, gentleness and kindness. Inviting them to rest their attention 'lightly on the breath' or bringing a 'gentle attention to emotions that move through them' or meeting their experience with a 'kind attention', highlighting that the quality of attention we are seeking is one of a friendly witness to our experience rather than a harsh, analytical observer.

In these ways, we highlight that mindful attention is something that can be intentionally directed and cultivated. This can enable students to step back from and observe their experience with more distance at times. At others, they can be encouraged to lean towards their experience, becoming more intimate with it.

In guiding students towards a more impartial witness presence explored in Section 1, it can be helpful to refer to exploring *the* body, *the* breath, *the* mind, *the* heart, softening tendencies towards defining these elements as 'I', 'me' or 'mine', which can make us prone to judging or defending rather than objectively observing them. That said, there are times when I will offer 'your body', 'your breath', etc., depending on whether a sense of connection feels more supportive than a quality of distance.

Normalizing experiences and celebrating differences

Misconceptions about yoga can result in students having expectations about what they *should* be feeling while practising. Our verbal cues might unconsciously feed into this, if stating that something *will* feel a particular way. This is where consciously inclusive and compassionate language comes in.

Over the years, I've heard of students persevering with practices that weren't appropriate for them because they were told it should feel good; their perception was that they were either doing it wrong or were meant to push through their discomfort.

We may have learned that *ujjāyi* breath is calming, forward folds are relaxing or Child's Pose is restful. While perhaps this is true for many, it won't be all. In our teaching, we can acknowledge that 'for some' these are the common responses while acknowledging that others' experiences may be different; neither is more nor less valid.

Through our guidance, we support students in noticing and naming what *they* are feeling rather than specifying what they *should* be experiencing. This gives students permission to both explore and validate their personal experience rather than questioning their truth if it varies from the 'norm'.

Rather than being definitive, we can offer suggestions, acknowledging that bodies might be relaxed, tight or tired, minds focused, dull or distracted. In normalizing different states, we highlight that the practice is about noticing. Students aren't wrong or failing in experiencing something different. In doing so, we empower students to trust, honour and respond wisely to their experience rather than ignoring, doubting or bypassing it.

Permission and possibilities

Similarly, using language that is invitational offers space to explore possibilities, promoting curiosity and self-inquiry, rather than suggesting certainties or preferences. Here are some examples:

- 'I invite you to'

- 'Feel free to explore'

- 'You might choose to'

- 'If it feels supportive'

- 'You're welcome to'

- 'As much as feels possible for you'

- 'Giving yourself permission not to'

- 'See how it feels to'.

These phrases highlight that the exploration is more important than a destination. Words and phrases such as 'perhaps' or 'maybe' offer autonomy to choose.

Of course, there will be times when we need to offer clear, explicit instruction to avoid injury and maintain safety. But in general, our choice of words can reflect that we don't *know* what a student's experience is nor how a practice will impact them. Even so, we can support them exploring and discerning what is right for them. Similarly, our alignment cues can allow for exploration and consideration of physiological differences rather than being definitive (unless safety is a clear issue).

Presenting options

Let's consider the language we use when presenting options and how this might impact students' perceptions of the practices, themselves and their choices. I prefer referring to 'options' or 'variations', as this highlights they are equally valid, whereas 'modifications' can create an impression of a perceived ideal that students are needing to vary from.

Similarly, presenting options from the most advanced to the simplest can imply that the first is the 'ideal', but if inaccessible there are 'lesser' variations that could be taken. Idealizing or referring to the 'full' or 'final' expression' of a pose can feed tendencies of striving, rather than students exploring and adapting as is most appropriate to them.

How different it can feel if instead we build options from the most accessible to more complex. Rather than labelling options as Level 1, 2 or 3, they are simply options 1, 2 and 3, highlighting that none are 'better' than the others. Similarly, when demonstrating, we might choose to remain longer in a variation that is more accessible than the most complex, conveying its equal validity with more physically demanding variations.

In presenting options, it can be helpful to frame choices positively. Consider how you might feel if the teacher demonstrates the most advanced expression of a pose and then offers 'if you *can't do* this', 'if this feels *too much*', 'if you are *struggling* with this', you could try X, Y or Z. Such language implies that we modify because we are struggling or lacking rather than being skilful in adapting.

How different it might feel to hear, 'If it felt *good* to use a prop on the other side, you might use it here' over, 'If you *needed* to use a prop on the last side…'. How much more empowering is it to help students discern which option feels more 'supportive', 'fitting' or even 'nourishing'; which variation enables their breath to feel most easeful or creates a feeling of spaciousness and stability. We might even encourage students to notice if they are being led by the wisdom of their body or being hijacked by the desires of their mind. After all, this is an important observation that they can carry with them off the mat into their everyday lives.

As more complex or demanding variations are offered, we can remind students that:

- 'deeper' physical form doesn't mean better and that attaining a certain shape doesn't make us happier, smarter, or kinder

- not being able to take a pose doesn't mean there is something wrong with us, simply that it's not the right version of the pose for us

- advancing in our practice is not about performing more complex or challenging shapes, but in deepening our capacity to listen to and adapt to our own needs, which will change daily.

When teaching in a group setting, we might acknowledge how lovely it is to see people taking different options, celebrating people making choices that respond to their needs.

Praising progression

Both in life and our practice, it is natural to wish for our efforts and actions to be seen, acknowledged and validated. Praise can stimulate feelings of reassurance, worth and belonging, sensing that we are on the right track.

Students understandably look to us as teachers for indications of what they are trying to move towards and where they are in relation to it. If we praise people only for their physical form, they will understandably assume that this is where 'success' lies in their practice.

When we consider broader definitions of progress explored earlier in this section, equally worthy of acknowledging and celebrating are wobbling bodies regaining balance with patience, focused attention, the tenderness of a gentle hand being placed on a hurting heart, the self-care practised when asking for an extra blanket or reaching for a prop, the self-awareness required when choosing to rest while others move.

During the Covid pandemic, as people practised online at home, often with little privacy and unfavourable conditions, my heart was frequently blown open with admiration as I witnessed examples of yoga in action – students patiently navigating enthusiastic pets; people committing to the stillness of *Śavāsana* as flatmates walked around (and at times over!) them, parents simultaneously practising while tending to their children. People often don't perceive such actions as signs of progress, but they are.

Such moments can trigger feelings of frustration and disappointment in students. Praising their practising calmness, kindness and steadiness amidst challenges can be illuminating, highlighting that progress isn't defined by our lives being peaceful but, in our finding greater peace within the realities we are living. One mother emailed after such a class to say how my acknowledging this enabled her to notice the ways in which the practice was helping her rather than focusing on how her environment was hindering her.

> **REFLECTION**
>
> – How might you broaden the praise you offer in your teaching?

Tuning into subtlety

It's easy for students to digest societal messages that 'bigger' is 'better', leading to perceptions that a 'powerful' practice contains bigger, stronger poses. Much of the power of these practices comes from our increasing capacity to tune into more subtle states. It is an advanced practitioner that can sense subtle shifts in the breath, the messages being offered by the gut, the undercurrents of emotions beneath their frustration. Tuning into subtlety enables us to discern the difference between pain and discomfort, a sustainable edge or pushing beyond it, breath that is nourishing or gasping. It enables us to discern when we are being led by the mind's grasping or the body's wisdom.

Our journey towards greater self-awareness understandably starts with noticing that which is most easily perceptible. Those new to yoga often need to feel something concrete (e.g., their feet on the floor) to feel something. Often, very mobile students seek strong sensation of stretch to be able to sense their body in space. This is understandable, but we want to be progressively increasing students' ability to tune into subtlety rather than always needing strong sensation to feel anything.

Noticing the more subtle elements of their experience highlights that yoga is more about tuning into subtle states than creating big shapes. We can invite students to open to parts of ourselves less frequently visited (e.g., the fingers, the space between their eyebrows or the pauses between the breaths, the spaces between the thoughts). It can be helpful to do this later in a practice when minds have begun to settle, rather than right at the start when they are often more scattered.

We can explain that tuning into subtlety helps us to detect the messages our body is offering (e.g., through our heart rate, our gut, our breathing) when whispering rather than only noticing when it is screaming. We can highlight how doing so within our practice enables us to become more attuned to the small things in life that so often go unnoticed (e.g., the warmth of the sun on our skin, a pleasant interaction) that bring feelings of joy and connection.

Spaciousness and silence

As important as the words we choose are, equally as precious are the moments of quietness we allow between them. At times, sufficient guidance is helpful to support a quality of presence, preventing minds wandering or wondering what they are meant to be 'doing' when 'nothing' is happening. However, equally important are the moments that we say nothing, offering space for our words to land, to be absorbed and most importantly for students to tune into *their* experience.

Sometimes, we can be so eager to 'give' students information or guidance that we forget that when their attention is drawn outwardly towards our voice, it is not tuning into their experience.

When inviting students to feel into something we might consciously take a few breaths after to allow space for presence. This can create a steady pace both for ourselves and those practising. The length of pauses will no doubt vary. Regular guidance might be helpful towards the start when everyday life is close by and minds are easily distracted, but we can keep our pace of speaking slow and spacious. Prolonged periods of silence may be more accessible towards the end when nervous systems have calmed and minds are more settled. This can be a lovely time to allow for extended periods of quietness, perhaps punctuated with poems or readings, letting their messages linger within the silence that follows.

In recent years, it has become more common for music to be played when teaching yoga. While I'm not suggesting that it is wrong, it can be helpful to consider how this might impact both ours and our students' capacity for mindful awareness.

I appreciate that is it a personal choice and that music may be central to your teaching. It can feel wonderful moving our bodies to music, particularly in unison with others. It can create feelings of joy and connection. Personally, I love it, but my yoga practice is not where I choose to do it. If you do choose to use music, you might explore offering some moments of quietness, perhaps at the start or end of practice. Space and quietness are rare for many people, not all moments of our lives need 'filling'.

For many years, I also played music, feeling that it helped to guide students into a state of calm that contrasted with the noisy soundscape of city living. As mindfulness became more central to my teaching, I became aware of its impact on my own ability to be present.

When I stopped playing music, I found the energy of the room felt more spacious. I could be more attentive to my students when not simultaneously considering a playlist. Initially, I felt more exposed without the music to hide behind, but soon realized it helped me to truly show up and be present. The pockets of quietness felt palpable and precious; they offered space for me to tune inwards and listen to my intuition, enabling me to be more responsive to myself and my students.

When attending classes where music is played, I find my attention often feels split between the teachers' instructions and the music playing. Music is subjective, what one person finds relaxing, another can find jarring. Even if we enjoy the music, we might consider how it impacts our capacity to tune into our internal experience.

REFLECTION

- How do you offer space for quietness and silence within your teaching?

Chapter 14

ANCHORS FOR AWARENESS

As we know for ourselves, minds wander; it is their nature. As well as offering guidance on how and where students place their bodies, offering regular suggestions on how and where to place their *attention* guides them towards a more mindful presence.

People's capacity for presence inevitably fluctuates as they practice. Our minds are likely to wander more when we first arrive to our practice but focus intently when we are standing on one leg!

There will be times when we sense that regular reminders would be supportive, and others when extended silences enable students to drop more deeply into their experience.

Guidance to 'notice your present moment experience' can feel somewhat broad, vague and easy to bypass. Offering navigation points beyond this, to specific elements of experience that students can tune into, can be helpful in maintaining interest and engagement.

In Section 1 we explored various pathways to presence; here, we will revisit them considering different ways to guide students towards them and points of inquiry to explore them.

Opening to the external environment

In opening to the external environment, we guide students to tune into their direct sensory experience, the sights, sounds and contact with the world around them. This can be a helpful starting point for some, for example, listening to sounds may feel more tangible than tuning into bodily sensations. If our inner landscape feels challenging or overwhelming, tuning into something external can provide a safer, more neutral option than the body or breath.

We might draw students' awareness towards:

- *The space around them:* Particularly when we first arrive on the mat, we can be consumed by thoughts, our attention narrowed and constricted. Opening to the space around them may allow students to feel held in a broader context, allowing for greater objectivity and perspective.

- *Their environment:* Tuning into their sensory experience – the sights, sounds and smells experienced in the moment. Doing so can help students notice how we respond internally to shifting external conditions. Even when conditions are less than ideal (I can think of the many times a car alarm has gone off when teaching in London), we can guide students to noticing how this impacts their inner experience, the thoughts that arise, the sensations in the body, offering a chance to practise equanimity.

- *Points of contact:* Drawing attention to the contact points between themselves and their environment (e.g., the ground, where air or clothing touches their skin) develops their capacity for proprioception, sensing where they start and end, how they relate to the space they are in. Again, for some, this can be more easily perceptible than more subtle internal sensations, so a helpful starting point.

We might ask students to inquire about the nature of their relationship with their environment, how easily they can allow themselves to drop into and be supported by the earth, whether they can soften and expand into the space around them.

Opening to the body

As we guide students to tune into their inner experience, we deepen their capacity for interoception, being able to listen to and decipher the internal messages of the body (e.g., sensing tension, ease, the heart beating, breathing, digestion). Doing so requires that we offer guidance not only on where to place the body in space, but on where to place *attention within the body*, and to become aware of what they notice when they do. I know for myself it is often only when someone invites me to feel into my jaw that I become aware of how much it is holding and its potential for softening; it is only when someone directs my attention to my side body opening that I sense the space offered and the sensation of the breath flowing.

Our guidance can support students in:

- *Noticing and naming sensations:* When so often lost in thought, people can become disconnected from their body and the messages it offers. Through our teaching we can guide students to noticing and naming physical sensations (e.g., engagement and release, warmth and coolness, vibrancy or dullness, even acknowledging places of numbness or where sensation is lacking). Doing so helps students to notice what tension and relaxation *feel* like, noticing *when* they are present, *where* they are experienced and *what conditions* contribute to them.

- *Mind/body connection:* Extending our guidance beyond alignment cues invites students to inquire into how something *feels*. It emphasizes that the external shape isn't the goal in our practice, but rather the vehicle through which we tune into our experience. For example, we can invite students to inquire into how it feels to root steadily into the earth in Mountain Pose (perhaps grounding), or to take up space in Warrior 2 (perhaps empowering), or to fold inwards in Child's Pose (perhaps quieting). Doing so supports students in sensing the intrinsic link between body, heart, mind.

  Similarly, we can help students become more attuned to their position within space, sensing the impact of our physicality on the different layers of our being. Noticing how the positioning of feet against the earth has a ripple effect through the alignment of the whole spine. Noticing shoulders that round, closing protectively around the heart, and how this impacts the quality of mind. Noticing how comfortable they feel taking up space or being small and whether this plays out in other areas of their life.

- *Broadening and narrowing attention:* Our experience of a practice can differ depending on how and where our attention is placed. At times, we can encourage a broad awareness; at others, a narrow focus. For example, if taking Warrior 2, a broad focus would guide students to noticing their whole body, inquiring how it feels to be grounded and open. Another time, we might invite them to narrow their attention towards one aspect, such as their connection to the earth, or the feeling of the heart opening which will offer a different experience. Another time, we might invite them to tune into where they sense stability or spaciousness, or where tension might soften.

- *Noticing habitual patterns:* When patterns of tension or alignment become normalized, we often fail to notice them (we might think of our shoulders living up by our ears). A simple thing such as changing the interlace of our fingers (or changing the fold of our arms or the cross of our legs) can raise awareness of how habitual we are with our bodies. Often, it is only when we do so that we realize how strange and unfamiliar it feels. Doing so highlights how much falls beneath our awareness and offers an opportunity to become more familiar with the unfamiliar and more comfortable with the uncomfortable.

- *Befriending bodies:* We can guide students to notice their *relationship* towards their body. Does it feel something to be dominated and shaped or embraced and embodied? When teaching, it is not uncommon to witness bodies in battle, shoulders straining and faces tensing, the breath held tightly. Supporting students in noticing their relationship to their body and cultivating a more compassionate one can be life changing. We will explore practical ways of doing this later.

It is important to be sensitive to the fact that people's experience of their bodies and their willingness or ability to connect to them will vary. For those new to yoga, tuning into the body can feel like navigating unfamiliar territory. For those living with chronic pain, the areas impacted might dominate their experience, drowning out perceptions of more subtle sensations. Injury or illness can impact our relationship to it, feeling somehow let down or betrayed by our body. Perceptions of 'normal' or 'ideal' bodies may leave some ashamed or disconnected from aspects of their physicality. For those who have experienced trauma, the relationship to the body can be complex, with certain practices potentially feeling unsafe or triggering.

As we guide students' attention progressively inwards, a common instruction is to close the eyes. However, for some, doing so can be anxiety inducing rather than calming. Feelings of safety for some are supported by maintaining awareness of the environment. Offering permission for both is helpful: highlight the potential benefits of closing the eyes (e.g., reducing external visual stimulation) for those for whom it is comfortable, while also offering permission to keep eyes open (suggesting a soft, steady gaze), should it feel more supportive.

While a path to healing can only come from reconnecting to these homes that we live our lives within, sometimes, the journey needs to be undertaken slowly, skilfully and sensitively. If you are working with clients who find it overwhelming, you may wish to deepen your learning about their condition or refer to a teacher with more experience.

Opening to the breath

The breath is central to our yoga practice. At times we guide students to shaping it, at others simply to observe it, but all the while it offers many opportunities to return to presence, feeling the life moving through us moment-to-moment.

Here, we might draw students' awareness towards:

- *Patterns of breathing:* We can guide students to noticing the nature of their breath, sensing its speed, depth, texture and location in the body, noticing helpful and unhelpful patterns and how it responds to internal and external factors. If students have difficulty connecting with the breath, they may find it helpful to feel it *against* something (e.g., the warmth of their hands on their body, or the contact of their body against a prop or the earth), creating sensations that are more palpable through the feedback offered.

- *Varying locations:* Again, we can guide students to both broadening and narrowing their perception; at times, sensing the whole-body breathing, or a specific area of the body that is opening (e.g., front, side or back body); at others refining attention to one area, such as the nose, the throat, the chest, or the belly (or simply wherever students sense the breath most easily). We may begin with that which is most easily perceptible and, over time, guide increased awareness of where it is more subtle (e.g., pelvic floor or back body).

- *Qualities imbued by the breath:* We can guide students towards exploring sensations associated with the breath (e.g., feelings of expansion, contraction or steadiness).We can invite curiosity about qualities offered by the inhalation (e.g., opening, receiving, spaciousness or enlivening) and those offered by the exhalation (e.g., calming, softening or releasing); the natural pauses between the breaths, and students' potential to tune into moments of stillness and non-doing.

- *Synchronizing movement and breath:* If teaching a flowing style of yoga, moving in sync with the breath (while maintaining qualities of slowness and steadiness) can support a focused attention as mind, body and breath unite. If teaching a group, it is understandable that we might set the rhythm, enabling people to move collectively. People's breath capacity will no doubt vary; what may feel an easeful breath count to us as a teacher may feel inaccessible to someone new to yoga. For this reason, we might offer times for students to move in alignment with *their* breath, normalizing that all our breath capacities will differ and offering them an opportunity to connect with and honour their own. Here, offering a repetition of a simple sequence (e.g., between 2 or 3 poses) can enable students to feel the power of dropping into the rhythm of their *own* breathing and moving in alignment with it.

- *Self-regulation:* While shaping the breath differs from mindful breathing, it offers valuable tools for self-regulating. Within *āsana* practice we guide the breath to becoming slow, smooth and steady, supporting a balanced nervous system where we feel alert but calm (each inhale stimulating the sympathetic nervous system, therefore, enlivening, each exhale stimulating the parasympathetic nervous system, therefore, calming). For many, their practice is the first time they've experienced their breath in this way and often offers insights into how the quality of our breath impacts our quality of mind. We can invite students to sense the breath like a barometer offering a gauge of their internal 'weather' system, whether at ease or pushing beyond their limits, both on and off the mat.

- *Relationship with the breath:* People's relationships to their breath varies. For many their practice offers a rare opportunity to even notice it. For others it offers a familiar source to steady and soothe us in difficult moments. If we have a history of anxiety or asthma, our relationship with the breath may be complex and fraught with judgements. Encouraging care and compassion as we meet the breath can be helpful. I like the idea of becoming more 'intimate' with the breath; such language suggests that we meet it with tenderness, care and curiosity rather than scrutiny. If we sense someone is forcing or over striving, we might encourage them to see the breath as something they are receiving, the body opening to the breath, rather than needing to 'do' the breathing.

- *The breath as a compassionate companion:* We can invite students to sense the breath's potential for soothing, particularly if we are in the midst of an intensity of experience. We can encourage a quality of tenderness with it, imagining its flow like a soft massage from the inside out, or we can intentionally direct the breath to a part of the body that is in need of care and attention. We might even suggest that students explore using each inhale to open to the present moment, and each exhale to bring acceptance and compassion towards it. We can acknowledge how the breath offers permission to take things one breath at a time, connecting to a quality of patient, steadiness when in the midst of intensity, reminding us that the nature of life is like the breath, it ebbs and flows, and as with all things, this too shall pass.

- *Mantra:* If the mind is strongly contracted or distracted some students might find using a mantra a helpful way of staying present with the breath. The *So Ham* mantra is considered a universal mantra that echoes the natural sound of the breath. Here, we silently say the sound 'so' for the duration of the inhalation and 'ham' (pronounced 'hum') for the duration of the exhalation. The translation of the mantra means 'I am that', with 'that' referencing pure consciousness, our true nature. The repetition of the sound (albeit silent) and intention, offering a more concrete focal point for the mind to rest on. Alternatively, simply offering the words, 'I am breathing in' on the inhale and, 'I am breathing out' on the exhale may feel more accessible to some.

Prāṇāyāma vs mindful breathing

While *prāṇāyāma* differs from mindful breathing in that it intentionally shapes the breath (to enliven, balance or calm our nervous system, often steadying the mind prior to meditation), practising mindfully acknowledges that one size doesn't fit all. For some *ujjāyi prāṇāyāma* supports mindful attention (as the mind rests on the smooth, ocean-like sound of the breath as the throat softly contracts); however, for others it can feel uncomfortable or unsettling. Encouraging mindful, compassionate presence enables students to acknowledge their experience and agency to use it or not depending on their personal experience.

In also offering moments of mindful breathing within our teaching (simply observing the breath's natural flow), we promote the power of allowing, accepting and even surrendering to the life that flows through us, without always needing to shape it. We might incorporate small pockets throughout our teaching or explore it for extended periods through a seated meditation (see Mindfulness of Breathing practice in Chapter 20).

Opening to thoughts and feelings

Our practice offers space to meet the whole of ourselves – bodies, minds and hearts. Thoughts and feeling will always form a part of our practice. Our intention isn't to clear our minds of thoughts, distract ourselves through movement or blissfully zone out from our feelings, it is to see ourselves more clearly.

Within our teaching we can guide students towards:

- *Observing mental/emotional states:* We can encourage students to step back and observe thoughts and feelings in the same way they would physical sensations, bringing curiosity towards them rather than immediately believing, feeling defined by or acting on them. In holding them more spaciously in our practice, we sense them more as 'mental events' that arise and pass rather than defining features of ourselves.

- *Noticing and naming:* At times, we might encourage students to notice and name the types of thoughts they are having (e.g., thinking, judging, planning) and emotions they are experiencing (e.g., joy, anger, frustration). Doing so can allow us to observe them more objectively and release the hold they have on us. As the saying goes, 'If you can name it, you can tame it'.

- *Mind/body connection:* We can guide students to notice how and where thoughts and feelings are felt in the body, whether frustration results in the body gripping or joy in the chest area softening.

- *Cultivating compassion:* We can encourage students to explore cultivating more supportive, encouraging qualities of mind (e.g., kindness, compassion, gratitude, equanimity). In a balancing pose for example, we might suggest that rather than gauging success in the body being stable, it can be found in working towards the heart/mind being calm and kind *amid* the inevitable wobbles.

Chapter 15

PROMOTING ATTITUDES OF MINDFUL AWARENESS

In Section 1 we explored the attitudes of mindful awareness. We will revisit them here, considering how we can guide students toward them. I find these a useful framework to draw on, noticing when someone might need a reminder to be patient, to soften judgements or bring more curiosity to their practice.

Beginner's mind

It is understandable that people come to yoga with expectations about both themselves and the practice. It is easy to slip into auto-pilot, particularly if we have taken a practice many times. How might we encourage students to cultivate a beginner's mind?

SUGGESTIONS FOR BEGINNER'S MIND

- *Language use*: We might suggest students feel into 'today's' body/heart/mind or explore a familiar pose with 'fresh eyes', 'as if for the first time'. We can encourage students to 'soften expectations', 'be open to possibilities' or be 'curious' and 'interested' in their experience.

- *Attitude:* Inviting students to consider a practice as something they are 'exploring' rather than 'doing'; considering not just 'moving' the body but 'meeting' it.

- *Encourage curiosity:* Guiding students' awareness towards more subtle, less explored elements of a practice (e.g., the air against their skin as they move, the breath in the back body). We might draw attention to less obvious elements of a pose, for example, when students are on their back circling their knees, inviting them to explore how the movement plays out in their upper body.

- *Variations:* Adding simple variations to common practices (e.g., varying the gaze, placement of the body, flow of breath) to encourage exploration and curiosity.

- *Asymmetry:* Inviting students to be attentive to our physical asymmetries and bringing a beginner's mind when taking an asymmetrical pose on the second side.

Non-judgement

Without careful attention, yoga settings can be breeding grounds for unhelpful judgements as students compare themselves to others or how they wish themselves to be. As teachers, we may be aware that one size doesn't fit all, but how can we convey this to students, encouraging them to soften judgements?

SUGGESTIONS FOR NON-JUDGEMENT

- *Modelling:* When we model this in offering a non-judgemental space as teachers, students sense permission to offer the same for themselves.

- *Noticing and naming:* Supporting students in noticing when unhelpful judgements arise and their impact on body, heart, mind and the tensions it can create.

- *Personal practice:* Highlighting that yoga is a personal practice supports students in respecting and valuing their unique needs rather than getting caught in comparisons. Offering options in a non-hierarchical fashion, emphasizes their equal validity.

- *Acknowledging and celebrating differences:* Recognizing the validity of different experiences (differences in physiology, breath capacity, life experiences) and so celebrating individuality.

- *Normalizing:* By acknowledging natural human tendencies (physical tension, minds wandering, strong emotions) judgements can soften when students experience them.

- *Encouraging:* When offering support, doing so in a way that is encouraging and constructive (rather than potentially construed as shaming).

Equanimity

Throughout their practice students will meet a range of 'feeling tones' of experience (pleasant, neutral and unpleasant). As we have seen, our brain's wiring draws us to desire and move towards that which is pleasant, bypass or ignore the neutral and pull away from that which is unpleasant. In cultivating equanimity, we encourage students to bring a balanced, caring attention to the full range of their experience, understanding that the nature of life is one of impermanence, there are ups and downs, nothing stays the same.

SUGGESTIONS FOR EQUANIMITY

- *Accessing steadiness:* Drawing attention to aspects of stability, whether through their connection to the ground, the flow of their breath or their gaze (known as *drishti*) can support students in tapping into a source of steadiness while simultaneously noticing the shifting nature of experience.

- *Welcoming:* Highlighting that our practice is a place to offer care and attention to the whole of ourselves (the parts that feel good, the parts that feel challenging, the parts we often fail to notice); that all are worthy of being seen and held, they are all welcome.

- *Pleasant experiences:* Supporting students in opening to pleasant experiences without striving for them.

- *Neutral experiences:* Guiding awareness towards more neutral experiences (e.g., the breath, heartbeat). Sensing how doing so enables us to appreciate elements of life that often fall beneath our awareness.

- *Unpleasant experiences:* Supporting students in noticing their relationship towards unpleasant experiences (pulling away from, ignoring or battling with it) and practising calmly exploring them. Meeting our 'edge' in practice (whether mentally or physically) offers an opportunity to do so, as does being with unfavourable environmental conditions (disruptions).

- *Impermanence:* Drawing awareness to the transient nature of experience (sounds arising and passing, sensations felt and fading, the breath inhaling and exhaling). Offering time to acknowledge shifts in body, heart, mind experienced at the end of a practice.

Patience

In this technological age of instant connection, with things done at the touch of a button, we might sense some students arriving to practice operating on high speed, seeking quick fixes or eager to 'progress'.

SUGGESTIONS FOR PATIENCE

- *Slowing down:* Highlighting that our practice offers an antidote to life's fast pace; it is a place where we have permission to slow down. We can acknowledge that bodies, hearts and minds open in their own time; it is not something that can be rushed nor forced but rather requires patience and presence.

- *Benefits:* Acknowledging that by practising slowly, gently and patiently we have time to tune into our experience, listening to and adapting wisely to our own needs, avoiding injury.

- *Personal practice:* Offering options in a non-hierarchical way, reduces perceptions that a 'better' experience is found somewhere else, therefore, encouraging students to be patient with where they are.

- *Injuries and illness:* While injury and illness are unpleasant, they hold the potential to support us in practising patience. I've often heard from students disheartened that health challenges have impacted their ability to practise in the way that they are used to. Without dismissing how hard this is, we might offer it as an opportunity to reframe perceptions of what 'advanced' practice is, and sense how meeting their new body with patience and acceptance is advanced yoga.

Non-striving

Striving is expected and celebrated in many fitness regimes. Some students may come to yoga with perceptions of 'no pain, no gain' or the aim to 'push beyond your limits'. For some striving has become the modus operandi in work and life and, therefore, seeps into practice. Non-striving doesn't mean complete inaction but rather practising in such a way that it is not dominated by grasping, either for physical forms or particular mental states.

SUGGESTIONS FOR NON-STRIVING

- *Practice vs perfection:* Highlighting that yoga is a practice, we are not seeking perfection. The attitude is one of exploration rather than performance or competition.

- *Less is often more:* Acknowledging that with less pushing and forcing for a particular outcome we often lessen strain and gain more peace of mind.

- *Language:* Avoiding language that suggests one option is 'stronger' or 'deeper' than another as this can be interpreted as better or more desirable. If we do feel these words are appropriate, we might stress that 'stronger' doesn't mean 'better', highlighting 'advanced' yoga is not about bigger or more complex shapes but rather deepening our capacity to be present and adapt accordingly.

- *Direction of travel vs destination:* We might acknowledge the difference between an intended direction we wish to move towards (e.g., to feel more caseful), over a goal (e.g., to touch our toes), which can feel like an end point we should strive towards or judge ourselves against.

- *Sustainability:* Exploring students' relationship to edge can be interesting and offer insights into patterns of pushing and striving (e.g., are they always pushing themselves hard for more). We might invite students to inquire if their relationship to their edge mirrors patterns in everyday life; does this impact their sense of sustainability or wellbeing in general?

- *Mind/body connection:* Guiding awareness to how striving manifests physically (e.g., faces straining, breath holding, muscles tensing) can increase students' awareness of its presence and impact. We can be particularly mindful of times when striving might manifest (e.g., extended breath retentions, physical binds in *āsana*) and draw attention to its presence and impact, reminding students that bigger doesn't mean better and that our practice should not feel like an endurance test.

Acceptance

As students practise with greater presence, they will inevitably meet elements that feel less than pleasant, whether in tight shoulders, busy minds, strong emotions or a car alarm going off outside. While part of our role as teachers is to offer practices that draw students towards greater ease and balance, part of this includes developing their capacity for acceptance. It is understandably easier to practise acceptance towards a tight hamstring than a breaking heart, but in building students' capacity to cultivate acceptance in one realm, we can develop their capacity to do so in others.

SUGGESTIONS FOR ACCEPTANCE

- *Befriending ourselves:* Explaining that acceptance is one way that we can learn to befriend ourselves. We don't have to wait until we are stronger, bendier, thinner or even calmer before we can accept and love ourselves.

- *Meeting difficulty:* Rather than ignoring, resisting, denying or immediately leaping into fixing less than pleasing feelings, we can encourage students to meet them mindfully and compassionately, accepting that, just for now, this is how it is.

- *Normalizing experiences:* Normalizing that our practice isn't only a space for love and light, but one in which we can open our hearts to *all* aspects of our lives; that tight or tired bodies, busy, distracted minds, happy or hurting hearts all form a part of our practice.

- *Celebrating individuality:* Acknowledging that the nature of being human is not one of perfection but rather an opportunity to explore and befriend our uniqueness.

- *Invitational:* Acceptance can be a big ask at times (it is understandable to want to resist or fix things that are painful). Offering 'as much as feels possible' to our guidance allows it to be presented as an invitation rather than a demand, something that we can nudge towards at a pace that feels manageable.

Trust

As teachers, our role is to be a supportive guide on students' journeys. While we might have ideas about what best serves them, we are not the expert on their needs or experiences, they are. An unhelpful (even dangerous) power dynamic is created when students feel they need to discount or bypass what they feel, because they assume that *we* are the authority on them and their practice.

This isn't to remove our responsibility towards students practising safely; we can be clear on how and why we feel a student should adapt or avoid a practice, enabling them to make informed decisions. But ultimately, we want to increase students' sense of agency and autonomy in the choices they make, helping them strengthen their capacity to listen to, trust in and respond to their intuition, their 'inner' teacher.

SUGGESTIONS FOR TRUST

- *Options:* In offering choices in our teaching, we encourage students to practise listening and responding to their intuition. For example, we might invite students to move between two poses (e.g., one active and one restful, or one open and expansive and another closed and protective) before inviting them to pause in the one that most meets their needs in that moment. Similarly, we can offer permission to adapt the level of intensity of a practice to their needs, for example by saying, 'this movement could be big or small, see what feels right for you'.

- *Intuitive movement:* Offering moments for students to move intuitively, listening and responding to their individual needs.

- *Acknowledging differences:* Acknowledging that people's experiences may differ. For example, we might offer a *mudrā* and note the intended impact (e.g., this *mudrā* is said to stimulate *prāṇa* in the lower lungs, so you may sense the movement of breath in the abdominal area) but acknowledge that people's experience may contrast from this. Doing so offers validity to students' experiences, rather than feeling they should distrust their perception if different.

- *Offering agency:* Acknowledging that students are the experts in their own experience and have the right to choose what is right for them. We can highlight that our guidance is a suggestion to explore rather than a rigid instruction to follow.

- *Self-regulation:* Guiding students to notice the messages the body offers when something *feels* intuitively right (perhaps a physical softening and opening) and when it *feels* wrong (perhaps a contracting and withdrawing). Encouraging students to discern when the body says 'yes' and 'no' and respecting its wisdom. In doing so, we empower students to be better able to discern their needs moment-to-moment, supporting *self*-regulation both on and off the mat (rather than needing our presence to facilitate it).

Letting go

Mindful awareness shines a light on patterns of holding (whether in a jaw clenching, a recurring thought or an emotion that we are gripped in).

Patterns of holding can block energy from flowing within us and prevent us from moving through the world with clarity and ease. Much of the practice of yoga is about letting go.

It can be helpful to remember that letting go isn't about pushing parts of ourselves away but rather involves letting go of our resistance or reactivity towards what we are experiencing, our judging, demanding or our attachment to things needing to be a certain way.

SUGGESTIONS FOR LETTING GO

- *Habitual holding:* When patterns of holding (whether physical, emotional or mental) are habitual, they often go unquestioned or unnoticed. Guiding students to become aware of them is the first step in letting go. We might alternate between poses that offer qualities of engagement and relaxation (e.g., inhaling shoulders up to ears and exhaling while releasing them) deepening students' capacity to recognize tension and ease and their impact.

- *Accessing support:* When talking of letting go, we might draw awareness to the support that students can release into. Whether that be the ground or props that they lean into, this can offer a sense of safety and support by letting go *into* something.

- *Invitational language:* When the idea of letting go feels strong, we might suggest students let go 'only as much as it feels OK to' or to explore 'softening the edges of what is holding', or 'letting be' instead of 'letting go'.

- *Shaking/sighing:* Offering practices that emphasize qualities of letting go (e.g., shaking out or letting out a big sigh). Sensing it in more concrete physical ways can lay the foundation to feeling it in more subtle states.

- *Exhale:* Each exhale offers a moment to practise letting go. The quality of our breath is so reflective of the quality of our minds that it's not uncommon for people who are tightly held (mentally and physically) to struggle to breathe out slowly and smoothly. Tuning into the exhale can offer interesting insights into our capacity to let go with ease, as well as a means of becoming more familiar and comfortable with doing so.

- *Compassion:* Acknowledging that, when letting go is not possible, we can be compassionate towards ourselves. Patterns of holding can be protective, and if the body, heart, mind are not ready to soften, we can meet this with tenderness and understanding rather than adding layers of judgements on top, which can increase tension.

Joy and gratitude

Given our brain's negativity bias, it is understandable that students' attention can veer towards perceived limitations and challenges rather than noticing and celebrating their capabilities. When not counterbalanced with acknowledging moments of joy, ease, strength or balance, our practice can become a place of dissatisfaction and frustration.

SUGGESTIONS FOR JOY AND GRATITUDE

- *Awareness of the positive:* Guiding students to notice positive qualities, such as strength, lightness, spaciousness, peace or ease; offering time to pause and stay with it, no matter how small it is, letting it be seen and felt, soaking it up.

- *Playfulness:* Encouraging elements of playfulness where we reconnect to a more child-like sense of joy in being in our bodies. Movement that feels intuitive, swaying and shaking can be lovely for this.

- *Gratitude:* Encouraging gratitude towards aspects of experience that nourish us, but which we often fail to notice (e.g., our breathing, our heart beating, our digestive system absorbing nourishment and letting go of what is not needed). Reminding students that our practice can be a place where we learn to enjoy our bodies, feeling grateful for their capabilities, allowing them to move and take up space as well as rest and lean into support. If we sense students' bodies appearing somewhat mechanical in 'doing' yoga, we might suggest they see how it feels to *enjoy* their body moving, breathing or resting.

Chapter 16

WORKING WITH PAIN AND DIFFICULTY

Our practice is a place to meet rather than escape our reality. In opening to our full experience, we are also teaching people how to open to and work skilfully with that which feels uncomfortable, painful or challenging. As we saw in Section 1, mindfulness offers us the steady, spacious foundation from which we can open to our experience. Kindness and compassion offer us the tools to work with, move through and grow from it.

As much as we might wish it otherwise, transformation and healing come from opening to the parts of us that are wounded, hurting and holding rather than bypassing or battling with them. This might be felt in the point of stretch of a tight hamstring, the frustration when wobbling or difficult emotions that rise to the surface when we allow space for them.

When working one-to-one with clients, we are likely to work on this layer of learning more deeply, finding out what is creating pain for them, and how it presents physically, mentally and emotionally; exploring what aggravates and alleviates it and the client's pattern of responding to it; exploring what needs space, what needs strength and holding, what needs acceptance and how we can bring compassion towards ourselves while experiencing it.

When teaching in groups, our work might be less in depth, but we can still acknowledge that this is a key aspect of the practice. We can normalize that pain and discomfort are a part of the human experience but that our practice offers ways to skilfully navigate it.

Many of us are more comfortable opening to/acknowledging physical discomfort rather than emotional pain. Learning how to be with unpleasant or strong bodily sensations, therefore, can be a useful place to start. When students are in a pose where they are likely to meet strong sensation, we can invite them to pause and notice their response to it.

- Are they adding layers of stories to it?

- Are they battling, pushing against or tensing around it?

- Is their response adding to or alleviating their tension?

- How is that reflected in their body and breath?

- How would it feel to explore their direct experience of it, allowing the steadiness of the breath to accompany them as they open to it?

- Does anything change or shift when being accepting and respectful of their experience?

As we support students in building their capacity to meet the edge of strong sensation (remaining present without exaggerating it, neither fuelling nor ignoring it, softening their reactivity towards it), we help them see that discomfort isn't solid and static rather it shifts and changes.

It is important to stress that this work should not feel like an endurance test. There is nothing to be gained from forcing people to remain in states that feel unmanageable, traumatizing or triggering. But rather, through our guidance, they can explore broadening their window of tolerance of what they can be present with. Doing so strengthens students' capacity to discern between the need for acceptance or compassionate action.

- Can they be and breathe with their experience?

- Can they offer space to gently investigate it?

- Does it require tending to (e.g., space or support, backing away from edge)?

- Is it more compassionate to shift the focus away from it (taking awareness to something neutral, such as sounds, contact with the ground or being soothed by Compassionate Breathing)?

What is key is building students' capacity to make choices based on clear seeing, rather than habitual patterns of reactivity.

As students learn to navigate discomfort within their bodies, we can highlight how the same tools support us when navigating it in our minds and hearts. Sometimes, students arrive to practice with mental or emotional pain at the forefront of their experience; at other times it arises unexpectedly. It is not unusual that when conditions of safety are created, as nervous systems calm and settle, as the busyness of the day's tasks subsides, that which we have pushed to the sidelines comes to the surface. We might notice an emotional response in a student, or simply sense a still point within the practice when it might be useful to acknowledge this. Normalizing this can be reassuring, particularly to those who are new to yoga who can be surprised and disconcerted when unexpected feelings such as anger or sadness arise. Again, we can acknowledge how normal this is and guide students to gently allow and explore their experience, without adding layers of judgement to it. For example:

- How is the pain expressed in the body? Perhaps fear sits like a knot in the belly, sadness like a contraction at the heart?

- Is it possible, for a moment, to gently lean in towards it, allow it and meet it with care and kindness?

Particularly when working one-to-one, taking time to explore such aspects offers valuable information on what our students are experiencing and how we can best support them through their practice.

This is where both kindness and compassion are so essential in our teaching – they enable students not to be stuck with their pain and suffering, but to find ways to work with and learn and grow from it.

Chapter 17

KINDNESS AND COMPASSION

For many, the concept of directing kindness and compassion towards ourselves can feel unfamiliar; the validity of our inner critic is often unquestioned; the belief that improvements are only achieved by pushing and punishing is prevalent.

Our yoga practice offers space to notice, challenge and change our relationship with ourselves to one that is more supportive. Care and kindness can be cultivated within our yoga practice through the way we move, the quality of our touch, our inner dialogue, the choices we take and our capacity to lean into support and rest.

A participant on my self-compassion course once fed back that the course felt 'like being wrapped in a warm blanket of acceptance and discovering that over the course you'd learnt how to take that blanket out into life with you'. How wonderful if we can show students how to create their own blanket of loving kindness and compassion so that they can carry it with them in their everyday life.

As we saw in Section 1, Kristin Neff defines the core components of self-compassion as mindfulness, common humanity and self-kindness. We've explored mindfulness in considerable depth, so let's explore the remaining two elements.

Common humanity

Environments that fuel feelings of comparison and competition can cause nervous systems to be vigilant and inner critics to be vocal. Similarly, perceiving our experience to be 'wrong' or 'not normal' can create feelings of shame and isolation. In contrast, promoting a sense of commonality, where people feel a part of a shared collective, can induce feelings of safety and belonging, which is calming.

SUGGESTIONS FOR COMMON HUMANITY

- *Inclusivity:* When teaching in a group setting, using the terms 'we' and 'us' conveys that we are practicing as a caring collective rather than being pitched against each other. Offering, 'those of us in need of restoring today might pause here, while those keen to move might continue to flow', highlights that whatever choice is made students are a part of, rather than veering from, a collective. Similarly, this conveys that we as the teacher sit within this circle of 'us', working with the same human experiences, rather than transcending them.

- *Normalizing experiences:* Acknowledging common human traits (e.g., minds wander, tensions gather, inner critics, bodies being asymmetrical) can make students feel connected rather than failing when experiencing them.

- *Collective support:* Creating a sense of collective support can help students feel connected to rather than in competition with fellow students. For example, in taking Tree Pose we might imagine roots reaching down into the earth, sensing how like groups of trees, our roots will inevitably intertwine, collectively supporting each other as we practice.

- *Loving Kindness*: Offering the Loving Kindness meditation (see Chapter 20) can promote a sense of our shared connection. When teaching in a group, we might simply offer these wishes of kindness towards each other or take the full practice where we extend it further towards all beings.

Kindness

As we have seen, loving kindness lies at the heart of mindful awareness. We encourage kindness when inviting students to meet their experience with presence, patience and acceptance, lessening patterns of denying, striving and judging. We encourage kindness when asking students to listen to their intuition, steering them towards self-care, balance and healing.

I remember once sharing a meditation in which I invited participants to 'meet themselves with kindness'. At the end, a student asked for clarification on what I meant, as they couldn't comprehend how this could be achieved. It was a great question and made me appreciate that while we understand what kindness is, we are often less sure about how to practically apply it. So, how can we incorporate this in more concrete ways into our teaching?

SUGGESTIONS FOR KINDNESS

- *Language:* Broadening our vocabulary around kindness can be helpful. Compassion isn't a commonly used term in everyday life, but people generally understand what it is to be 'gentle', 'warm', 'caring', 'tender', 'loving' and 'friendly'. We can thread these terms within our teaching, inviting people to bring a 'gentle' attention towards their breath, feeling the 'warmth' of their touch, inviting touch to feel 'tender and caring', meeting themselves in a 'loving' and 'friendly' way, 'kindly' placing a foot into position, taking options that feel most 'supportive'. Similarly, words such as 'encouraging', 'offering', 'gathering' and 'guiding' have a softer tone than those of 'placing', 'taking', 'doing' or 'using'.

- *Kindly awareness:* We might suggest students meet themselves with a kind awareness, as if viewing themselves with kind eyes and a soft heart, reminding them that their practice isn't a space to analyse, demand or judge but rather space to gently open to themselves.

- *Terms of endearment:* Small words can have a significant impact. Referring to our 'dear mind', 'dear body', 'dear heart' can be powerful, sensing tenderness towards these different layers of ourselves, encouraging students to meet and respond to them as they might a dear friend.

- *Noticing inner narratives:* Drawing students' attention to the nature of their inner narratives can help them notice if they are supportive and encouraging or harsh and critical. Encourage students, at times, to consciously talk to themselves (albeit often silently) in more supportive and kind tones and terms, while noticing the impact. Perhaps there are some words of kindness that they could do with hearing today – invite them to say them silently to themselves.

- *Self-care:* Encouraging students to make choices based on self-care over performance; meeting themselves with kindness rather than forcing (which can leave us prone to injury); adjusting 'traditional' alignments (e.g., gazing at the top hand in *Trikoṇāsana*) if an alternative gaze (e.g., at the wall or floor) feels more appropriate and avoids straining.

- *Compassionate breathing:* We might suggest imbuing the breath with a quality of kindness; that, as it smooths and steadies, it becomes soothing, like a gentle massage from the inside out. This could be directed to anywhere that particularly needs tending.

- *Compassionate smile:* Incorporating the image of a compassionate smile, one that is soft, gentle and can hold whatever we are feeling in kindness (not a huge beaming smile that feels forced or false). We might use this in a meditation or when in *Śavāsana,* visualizing or sensing the smile as an external force shining down upon us, before placing the image of the smile within our own lips, eyes or heart, sensing how it feels for these parts of us to be held in kindness. At other times, we might encourage students simply to sense the possibility of a gentle, kind smile as they hold a pose, noticing how its essence plays out through the body, heart, mind. In the words of Tara Brach: 'When we meditate with the spirit of a smile, we awaken our natural capacity for unconditional friendliness'.[1]

- *Support:* When offering the option to use support (e.g., sitting on a chair for meditation or using supportive touch to help a limb into position), we can frame this in the context of self-care. We might suggest offering the foot 'a kind, helping hand' if it doesn't come all the way on its own to ensure it is framed in the context of practicing kindness rather than being compromised or failing.

- *Comfort: Śavāsana* can be a lovely practice to encourage students to practise offering themselves care, reaching for that which makes them feel comfortable, warm and supported. I often suggest that students imagine tucking themselves up in the same way that they would a loved one. Sometimes, this can offer insights into how differently we treat ourselves and permission to offer ourselves the same care and attention as we might extend to others.

Connecting to our hearts

In the English language our hearts have often been linked to emotional states of love and loss. We describe people as being 'open', 'closed', 'warm' or 'cold' hearted. We recognize times of feeling 'light' or 'broken' hearted.

Within the yoga model of the *cakras* (energetic centres within the subtle body), *anāhata cakra* – often referred to as the 'heart centre' – is located in the chest area (the whole chest cavity rather than restricted to the organ of the heart). It is here that we feel the expression of qualities of unconditional love, care and compassion. It is where we feel the impact of grief, hurt and loss. These differing emotional states are expressed in our physicality. When we are joyful, we stand taller as we meet the world, our chest opens, our breath is more easeful. When we are sad, our shoulders slump, our backs round, our breath is restricted as we close protectively around the heart centre.

SUGGESTIONS FOR CONNECTING TO OUR HEARTS

- *Āsana:* Both in movement and stillness certain poses can draw attention to patterns of openness and holding within the heart space. We often think of 'heart-opening' poses as backbends that open the front body, but equally as important is allowing freedom of movement in the sides and back. We want our hearts to be able to open to the world *and* protectively soften inwards towards ourselves. What we wish to avoid is being stuck in one mode. If we sense that someone is caught in a pattern of closing, moving slowly between opening and closing (e.g., the openness of Cow Pose and the protective quietness of Child's Pose) offers a gentle way for the body to sense the potential for change, while being offered the safety of returning to its familiar, protective state when needed.

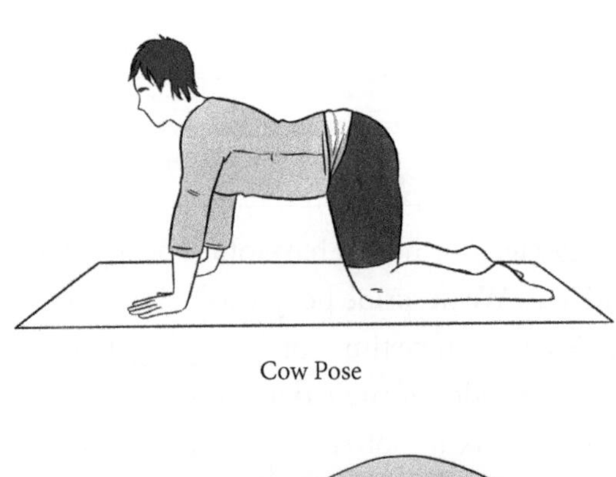

Cow Pose

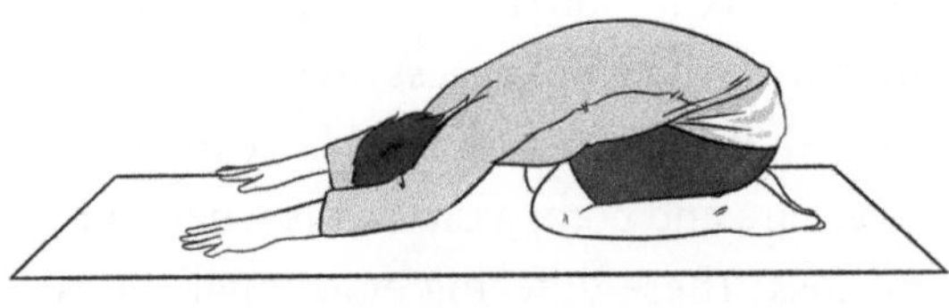

Child's Pose

- *Breath:* Guiding students to notice the expression of the breath offers insights into whether energy flows with ease or feels limited in the chest area. Again, in encouraging the breath to become smooth and soothing, we can invite students to imagine the heart-space being nourished and opened by the inhale and soothed and softened by the exhale. If helpful, placing the hands onto the chest can offer a more easily perceptible sense of the breath here.

- *Rest:* One of the kindest things we can offer ourselves is rest. Restorative yoga can be a lovely way for students to sense that opening our hearts needn't be rushed, nor involve pushing or forcing, but rather creating the conditions of safety and support that allow it to open when ready. Leaning into the support of props and being covered with the softness of blankets can offer conditions to feel soothed, calm and held.

   Again, small, progressive steps are most supportive. If someone is experiencing deep sadness, placing them in an extreme backbend for extended periods could potentially feel jarring, exposing or making them feel vulnerable. Instead, we can start small and deepen progressively if it feels necessary.

   For example, we might begin by opening the front of the chest with a simple, subtle backbend. In the option below, a strip of blanket is placed lengthways along that mat, the top end placed on a flat block. The student then can lie with their spine over the blanket, their head supported by the blanket and block to open the chest gently.

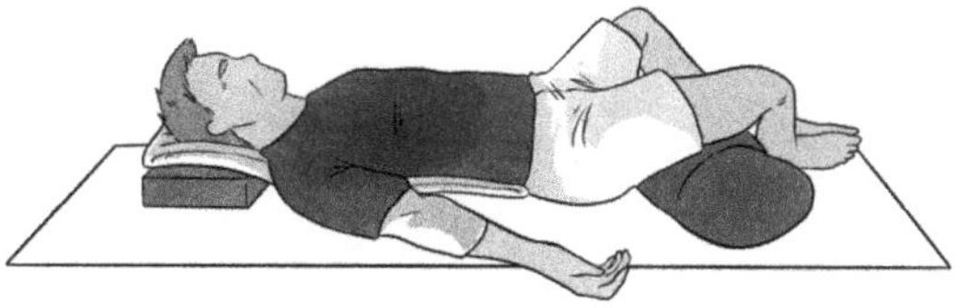

Gentle Restorative Backbend

When appropriate, a deeper sense of opening could be created by using a bolster to lift the chest. Here, a flat block is placed under the seat to prevent over-arching the lower back. A folded blanket is placed under the head to allow for the chin to be slightly lowered (which promotes stimulation of the parasympathetic nervous system), but a range of adaptations could be created to support students' individual needs.

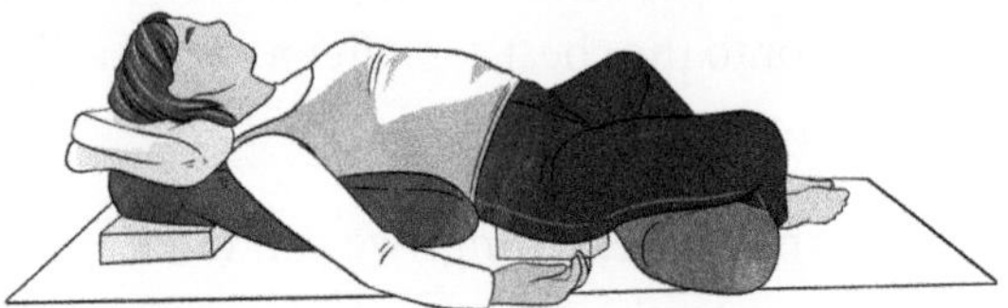

Deeper Restorative Backbend

Equally as supportive can be offering restorative poses that open the chest in all directions, not only the front, but also the sides and back of the ribcage.

In the side-opening restorative pose, bolsters are used (but could be replaced by pillows or rolled blankets, depending on body dimensions) to allow the side of the chest to open. The pose would be repeated on both sides. For those with shoulder restrictions, blocks may be used under the hand on the extended side to avoid straining (as shown here) or the hand could be placed directly on the bolster. If more comfortable (it can depend on body dimensions), a folded blanket can be placed under the hips to reduce the distance between the ground and the bolster. A reminder that we are looking for ease and relaxation in restorative poses and not strong sensations of stretch (which keep the nervous system more activated).

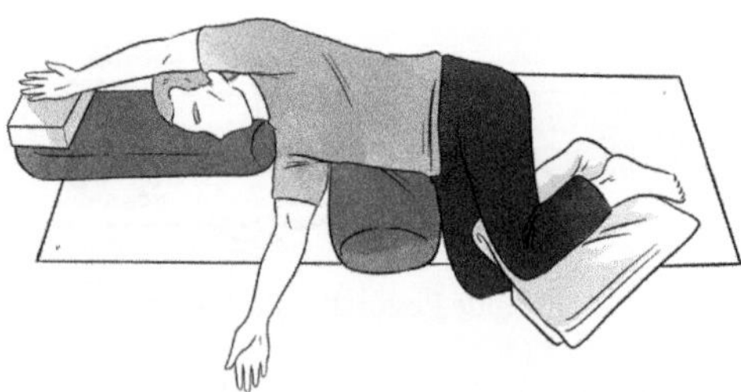

Side-Opening Restorative: Opening the sides of the ribcage (taking on both sides).

In this version of Restorative Child's Pose, a bolster is placed between the legs with the torso softening into it, the head turned to one side. If a student requires more height a block (or more) could be placed under the top end of the bolster. If the student finds discomfort in the ankles, a rolled up blanket can be placed under them. If there's discomfort in the knees, a folded blanket or block could be placed between the thighs and calves. Alternatively, Front Lying *Śavāsana* (see Chapter 20) may provide a more comfortable variation.

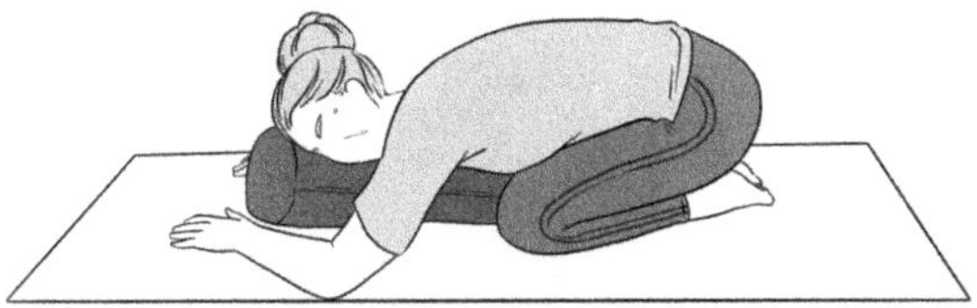

Restorative Child's Pose: Opening the back of the ribcage.

- *Mudrās and compassionate gestures*: These can be a lovely way of encouraging students to notice, connect to and tend to their hearts.

  - *Padma mudrā: Padma* means lotus and so this *mudrā* is like a lotus flower that we hold close to the heart centre. It can be helpful to begin in *Añjali mudrā* with palms touching; then, keeping both thumbs connected and both little fingers also, the other fingers open outwards like a blossoming flower. For me, the image of the lotus flower conjures up qualities of strength (as it roots deeply into the soil beneath the water), beauty and vulnerability with its delicate petals. Such qualities feel fitting for connecting to our hearts.

    The openness of *Padma mudrā* reminds me of a cup-like container. At times, I will offer this as a meditation, inviting students to consider what their heart needs to be topped up with (e.g., strength, joy, contentment, ease); then, imagining breathing this in, filling the cup with each inhale and letting its contents be absorbed deep within them with each exhale.

Sometimes, I'll combine *Padma mudrā* and *Añjali mudrā*, imagining the cup filling on the inhale as we take *Padma mudrā*, then sensing ourselves sealing this nourishment within as palms touch in *Añjali mudrā* on the exhale. Alternatively, we can imagine directing this kindness outward, imbuing the heart with kindness as we inhale with *Añjali mudrā*, then imagine extending this kindness outward to the world as we open the palms into *Padma mudrā* on the exhale.

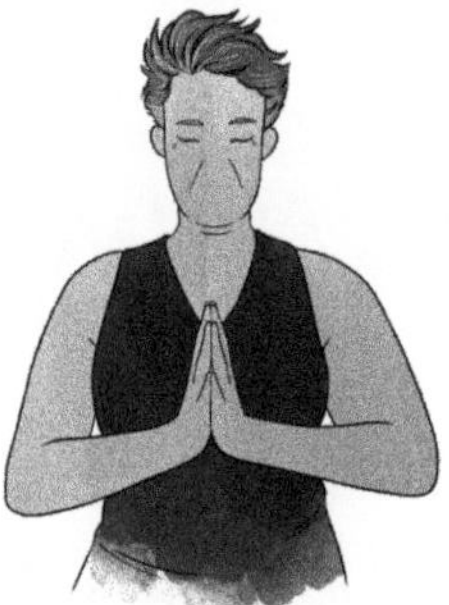

Añjali Mudrā

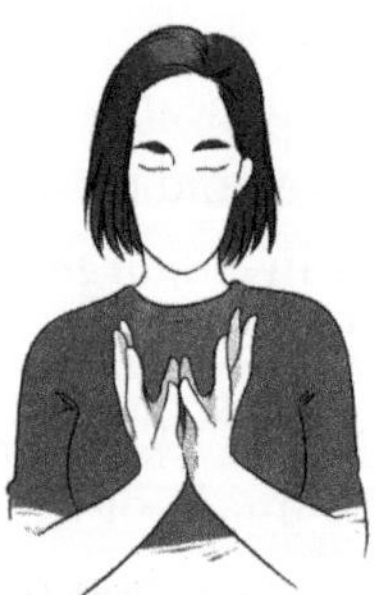

Padma Mudrā

– *Palms against the chest*: Simply placing one or both palms on the chest (one palm on top of the other) helps us connect to ourselves in a caring manner, sensing our capacity to be both the giver and receiver of care.

The placement of the hands offers greater sensory feedback to explore whether the heart is open or closed, whether the breath flows with ease or feels restricted. We might inquire whether the palms feel rigid or soft, whether we can feel and receive their warmth, whether we can sense our breath or even heartbeat under our palms. Particularly if the body is holding patterns of pain or difficulty (whether physical or emotional), incorporating caring touch can help students explore feelings that might be uncomfortable or unpleasant, while simultaneously meeting them with care and tenderness.

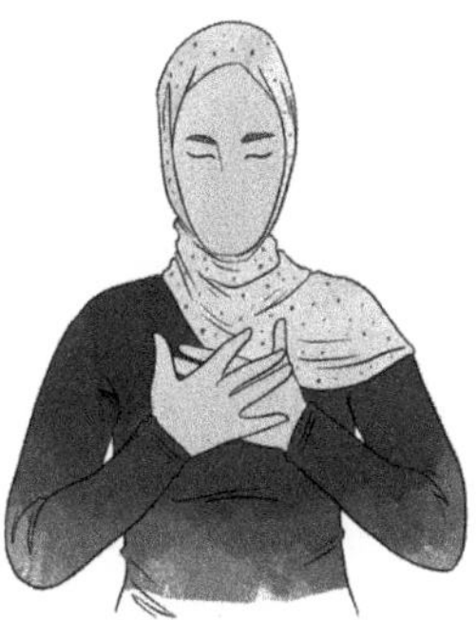

Hands on Heart

—   *Palm over fist:*[2] A compassionate gesture offered by Kristin Neff is to make a fist with one hand and place this at the centre of the chest, then to wrap the other palm over the top. This simple variation from the one above can have a surprisingly different impact. For me, the firmness of the fist, wrapped in the softness of the palm, cultivates a sense of inner strength. At times when we need to draw on a courageousness of heart or a fiercer quality of compassion, this can be a powerful gesture.

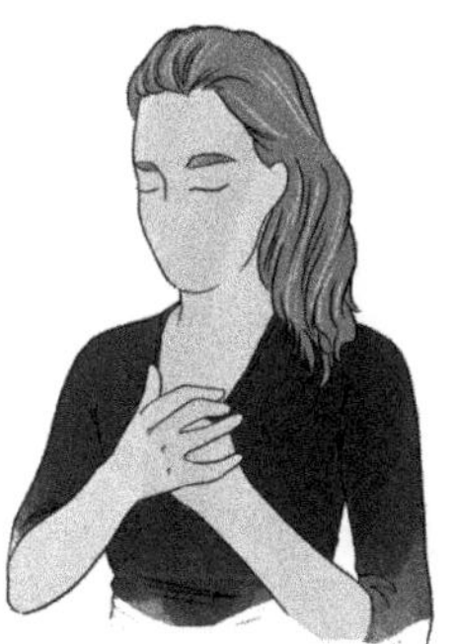

Palm over Fist

– *Vajrapradama mudrā (Gesture of Unshakeable Trust):* This *mudrā* is said to open *anāhata cakra*, directing the breath, awareness and *prāṇa* to the chest area. It encourages qualities of openness, confidence and trust in ourselves and life. Here, we interlace the fingers with the thumbs outstretched and place the palms on our chest. I find it encourages a sense of openness as the chest spreads under the hands and a sense of strength and connectivity as the fingers interlock.

We might use this within a seated meditation or incorporate it within an *āsana* practice. I find this a lovely *mudrā* to use while connecting to the heart and listening to whether there are any words it needs to hear and then offering them to ourselves.

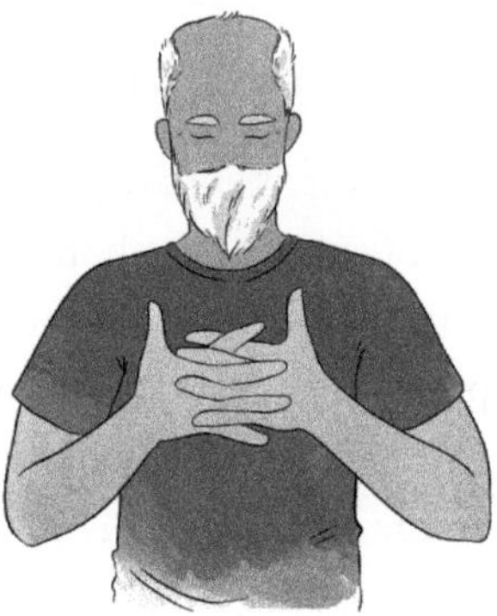

Vajrapradama Mudrā (Gesture of Unshakeable Trust)

– *Hand to heart, hand to earth:* This simple, seated gesture invites us to tap into qualities of kindness and steadiness. Here, one palm spreads softly against the chest, the fingertips of the other hand are connected to the earth. If needed, you might place a block or blanket under the hand that connects to the ground to ensure that the spine remains tall rather than leaning to the side to maintain connection.

I use this gesture in a variety of ways.

› Offering it at the start of a practice, as a means of tapping into qualities of care (via the hand on heart) and steadiness (tapping into the steadiness of the earth via the hand connecting to floor). Sensing these as foundational qualities for practice in body, mind and heart.

› Inhaling connecting to a feeling of drawing steadiness from the earth. Exhaling connecting to a sense of kindness towards self.

› Inhaling connecting to feelings of warmth and care at the heart. Exhaling, imagining sending care outwardly towards others or the world via the connection to the earth.

This can offer an interesting variation of the Loving Kindness meditation, for students who find it helpful to have a more physical reference point when offering kindness inwardly and externally.

› When practising in a group, it can be a lovely way to practice both giving *and* receiving kindness. As the practice is taken collectively, we can imagine extending care outwards as we exhale and receiving the care that others have offered as we inhale, and in doing so deepening feelings of connectivity with those we practise with.

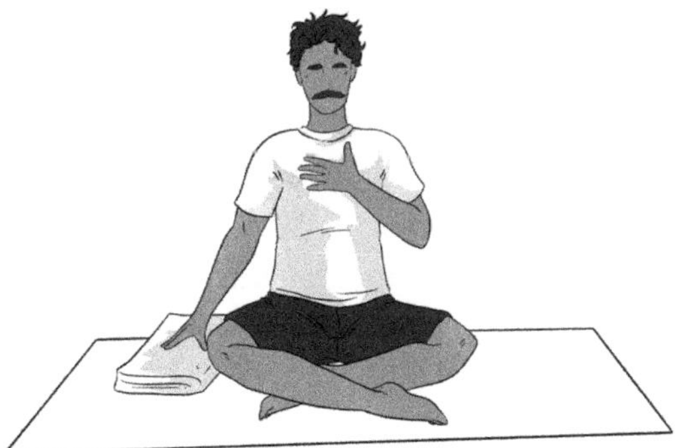

Hand to Heart, Hand to Earth

- *Conversing with the heart:* For those living in cultures that place greater value on intellectual thinking over feeling, the concept of listening to our hearts can be unfamiliar, but in the words of

Jack Kornfield, 'It is possible to speak with our hearts directly. Most ancient cultures know this. We can actually converse with our heart as if it were a good friend.'[3] When I choose to do so, I'm often struck by the contrasting content and tone offered by my heart and head. My head is often more eager to play the role of the inner critic, seeing problems to be fixed and dangers to be avoided. My heart offers more of a compassionate companion, willing to see the bigger picture and hold tenderly whatever I'm experiencing.

Within our teaching we can offer moments where students can quietly listen to this heart-felt wisdom. We might inquire, 'If there were something that your heart needed to hear just now, what might it be?', or 'Drop into your heart and ask in what small way might you offer care towards yourself in your week ahead?'. Adding the term 'might' is intentional, as it encourages us to consider the question from our intuitive wisdom, which is open to possibilities, rather than our analytic mind that tends to seek 'correct' or 'definitive' answers. Given that listening to the heart may be unfamiliar to many, we can emphasize that it is OK if nothing arises, but there is still benefit in offering space to curiously listen. I find students are often very receptive to this and, sometimes, surprised by the clarity of the words they hear in response; for example, being told they are enough, precious or worthy of caring for.

- *Courage:* If we sense students' resistance to self-compassion, considering it weak, soft or fluffy, we might highlight that it takes strength to allow hearts to open, courage to meet our present moment experience with tenderness. We can invite students to feel this in their physicality, when sitting placing one hand on the heart centre and one on the belly, noticing how the gentle strength in our centre (with abdominal muscles lightly engaging on the exhale) supports the chest in opening; that there is a relationship between strength and softness, space and support. That rather than them being opposing qualities, they are complimentary ones, and we benefit when they co-exist.

Self-soothing touch

As we saw in Section 1, our capacity to self-soothe supports us in self-regulation, helping to steady and calm ourselves when thrown off balance. We've already explored some self-soothing techniques in this section, but here let's specifically consider self-soothing touch.

We often think of caring touch as something we do in conjunction with another, but supportive *self*-touch enables us to become both the giver and receiver of care. Part of the power of self-touch is that rather than *thinking* about being kind to ourselves we viscerally *sense* it. For many, particularly those new to self-compassion, well-worn inner narratives of self-criticism can create resistance or scepticism when offering words of kindness towards themselves; the inner critic leaping in with, 'hold on, I'm really not *sure* about this!'. Touch, however, stimulates a more embodied response, tapping directly into our nervous system, as if bypassing our intellect that can question it. I have felt this in myself and had this fed back to me by students.

Incorporating supportive, caring touch into our teaching can offer students insights into how they meet themselves. Just as inner narratives can be critical, students can become aware that they physically connect with their body in a way that is detached or mechanical rather than caring. A student once commented after class that using caring touch made her realize how often she met herself from a place of demanding and pushing and how different it had felt to connect with herself in a manner that felt kind.

SUGGESTIONS FOR SELF-SOOTHING TOUCH

- *Stroking/massage:* Incorporating stroking and gentle massage into our teaching can increase students' perception and caring connection towards different parts of the body. Sometimes, I will offer time at the start of practice to bring caring touch to the face and head. Here, we could invite students to: gently run their fingers through their hair or scalp, encouraging the quality of touch to feel soft and caring, as if soothing a small child;

stroke the brow, as if soothing places that have furrowed from concentrating; circle fingers around temples; massage around the jaw to release tension here. We might invite them to stroke down the side seams of the neck or give the shoulders a gentle squeeze encouraging students to tune into how caring touch feels and how the mind, body, breath respond to it.

We can use this within an *āsana* practice. For example, in a seated side bend we might gently stroke the side body, before pausing with the palm in one place sensing the breath under our palms, soaking up the warmth of our hands.

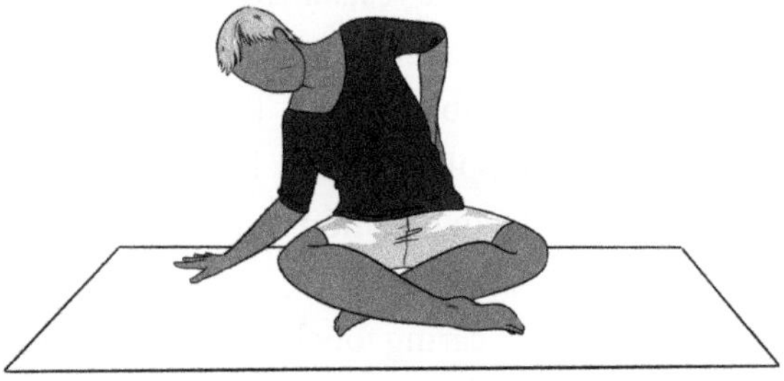

Seated Side Bend with Touch

As we flow between poses, we might incorporate caring touch; for example, gliding our hands up and down our legs (either when seated or incorporating it into a standing flow). When opening the chest, we might invite one hand to stroke along the opposite arm and across the heart before reaching to the sky.

The quality of being massaged can extend beyond our hands. For example, in Child's Pose we can invite students to sway the forehead slowly side to side against the mat or a block, imagining massaging the brow and soothing our often-busy mind. When on the back, hugging knees to chest, we can encourage gently rocking side to side sensing the spine being massaged against the ground. Here, our guidance can create a shift in intention from one of simply 'moving' to one of caring and soothing.

- *Generating warmth:* To increase the perception of caring touch we might invite students to rub their hands together initially, generating a quality of heat, so that when placed on the body, we can sense that body part soaking up the warmth offered by the hands. I often like to offer this over the eyes, which may have spent days on screens, or over the kidneys, imagining the adrenal glands that sit on top being soothed after a busy day. Similarly, we might invite students to place their hands wherever they feel the warmth and care is most needed that day.

- *Hugs:* Virginia Satir, a family therapist, is quoted as saying, 'We need 4 hugs a day for survival. We need 8 hugs a day for maintenance. We need 12 hugs a day for growth.'[4] If this is true, most of us need more hugs. During the lockdowns of the Covid pandemic, when so many were deprived of caring touch, self-hugs became a regular feature of my online classes, and their presence has continued since. Whether taken standing up, sitting down, on our backs or on our side, as students wrap their arms around themselves, they can directly sense the power of tenderly holding themselves.

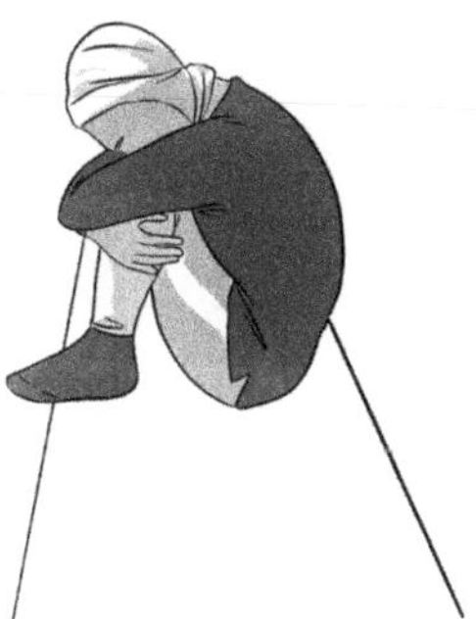

Seated Hug

At times I've suggested that students imagine how the quality of their touch might change if they imagined they were hugging someone else. Students have sometimes commented that this simple suggestion resulted in their body softening more, their breath deepening and their connection feeling more caring, highlighting the contrast between how we offer care to ourselves and others.

We can incorporate self-hugs within flowing sequences

alternating between poses that open the heart to the world, and ones where the arms wrap around ourselves. We might then invite students to stay in whichever one feels most needed for a few breaths, highlighting that, some days, it feels good to be open to the world and, at other times, to fold inwards towards ourselves.

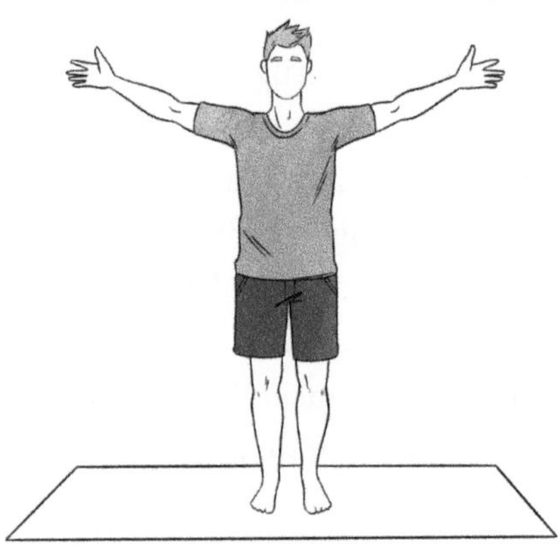

Standing Arms Open

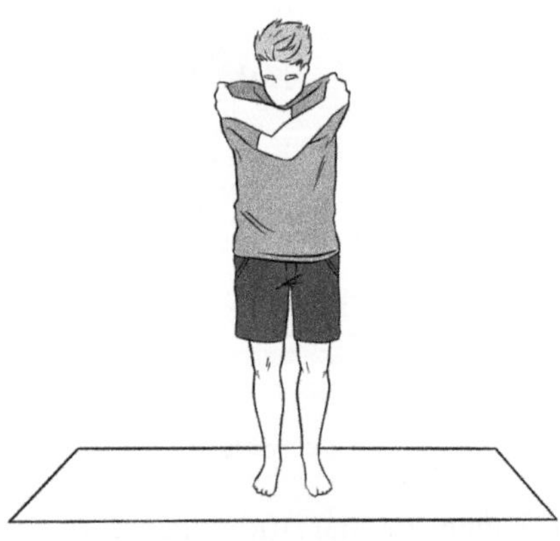

Standing Hug

We might also bring this into restorative yoga, guiding students to notice how it feels to be hugging the bolster. Sometimes, I invite students to place the bolster lengthways on their chest when lying supine and wrap their arms around it, noticing the response in body, heart, mind to this 'virtual' hug.

Once again, it is worth acknowledging that we are all different both in our innate make-up and our life experiences. While self-touch may feel safe and soothing for some, for others, it may not and so offering permission to participate without enforcing it offers students agency to choose.

REFLECTION

- In what ways do you build kindness and compassion into your teaching?

Holding space for emotional responses

Kindness and compassion are often perceived as 'soft' or 'gentle' qualities, but they can require strength and courage to practice. Our defences offer a protective barrier and softening our armour needs to be undertaken slowly and sensitively rather than ripping it off like a plaster.

Opening our hearts to ourselves can be emotional, particularly when we've not learnt how to do so. That first time I practised self-soothing touch on retreat, I was surprised to find tears unexpectedly flowing. This can be common when we soften our edges and touch in on places in need of healing and holding. In sensing the potential safety of being seen and held, emotions that have been supressed can rise to the surface. As we explore meeting ourselves with care and tenderness, feelings of grief can arise as we recognize how long we have denied ourselves this.

As teachers, we might find tears a welcome visitor, seeing them as an emotional release of something that was blocked. Some students, however, can be surprised, embarrassed, or even feel ashamed by, their presence, as well as confused in not being able to pinpoint where they have stemmed from.

When students have a strong emotional response, it can be helpful to first acknowledge what this brings up in us. Do we feel uncomfortable or unsure of how to respond? Does it bring up sadness in ourselves? Can we bring self-compassion to that? Do we feel an urge to leap in, offering comfort or support?

While the urge to comfort someone (offering caring touch or a tissue) comes from a compassionate place, it can also unconsciously convey that tears are a problem to be fixed, and we wish for them to stop. Holding space steadily and compassionately, without leaping into action can show students that we are comfortable in the presence of emotional responses, there is nothing to be ashamed of.

In a group setting, we needn't single anyone out but might acknowledge that unexpected emotions or tears are a common and normal response. We might add that we needn't know or analyse their origin, we needn't judge ourselves, but rather understand that it can be the body's way of releasing things that it has been holding. At the end of class, we might gently check in with the student without placing pressure on them to expand on their experience, but let them know we are there should they have any questions.

In some situations, if a student appears to be overwhelmed or in a pose that could feel exposing (e.g., lying on the back), offering a Side Lying *Śavāsana* can offer a sense of privacy, protection and support while strong emotions are present (see Chapter 20).

REFLECTION

- What comes up for you when someone has an emotional response to a practice?

Chapter 18

PACING AND PAUSING

Going slow

In the words of Donna Farhi, 'If we were to do nothing else in our spiritual practice but reduce our accelerated pace, the world would be transformed overnight.'[1] The speed at which we move through life impacts the quality of awareness that we bring to it. In slowing down our pace, we dial up our capacity to tune into our experience.

As mindfulness became more central to my teaching, the pace of my practice and teaching naturally slowed. I love teaching flowing sequences (and feel they hold value when many people's lives are sedentary), but offer them at a speed that allows students to practise mindfully. I find myself increasingly drawn to more still, meditative practices, such as yin and restorative yoga, that offer greater time for reflection and inquiry.

Practising slowly enables us time to tune into our embodied experience; to feel our connection to the ground, places of ease and tension, where the breath is flowing, the impact that a practice is having; how we would benefit from adapting. It enables our practice to be a space for exploration rather than another thing we are 'doing'. It stimulates the parasympathetic nervous system where minds calm and we can access our rational and more intuitive wisdom.

As teachers we can drop in points of inquiry that help students notice their relationship to speed, for example:

- What happens when they slow things down?

- Does it feel delicious or excruciating?

- How does speed play out in their wider lives?

This is all useful information that we can guide our students towards noticing.

There will, of course, be times when our practice might be intentionally fast to stimulate a particular effect. This isn't bad, but there is a difference when doing so with awareness, acknowledging its impact rather than speed being an unconscious habit that dominates our life and practice.

Slowness can be a useful precursor to stillness. Going from 90 mph to zero quickly can be unhelpful and uncomfortable. Many of us need to decelerate first, otherwise our body is still, but our mind is racing full throttle which feels far from peaceful. As slowness becomes more comfortable, stillness often feels more accessible.

REFLECTION

Take a moment to reflect on how speed plays out in the classes that you teach.

- Do you fall into delivering practices at speed because you think it is what students want or because you feel it is what they need?

Pausing

Offering moments to pause within practice helps students sense the power and importance of simply opening to our experience as we find it, without always needing to shape it. It offers space to sense the *impact* of a practice – in physical sensations, the quality of energy flowing through the body, the nature of the breath, the quality of mind and heart. It offers points to reconnect with intentions or motivations for practising and whether they are practising in alignment with them.

Such moments can offer interesting points for inquiry, noticing their relationship to pausing, whether it feels a welcome relief, unfamiliar or challenging. This can vary day-to-day but offers valuable information about how they are balancing being and doing.

Offering pauses requires us as teachers to be comfortable in creating spaces that don't need filling. It is easy to be drawn into wanting to 'give' more (more poses, more practices, more guidance) so that students are getting the most from our offering. It can be helpful to remember that often giving less offers space for students to feel and receive more, emphasizing the importance and power of moments of simply being.

If we find creating pauses challenging within our teaching, we might explore our own relationship to stopping. Often, the more we are comfortable in pausing ourselves, the more comfortable we become in holding space for others within them.

REFLECTIONS

- In what ways do you build pauses into your teaching?

- What is your own relationship to moments of pausing? Do you feel comfortable with them or feel drawn to filling them?

Chapter 19

OFFERING SUPPORT

Assisting students

Over the years, I've had mixed experiences of receiving hands-on assists. There have been times when I've enjoyed my body being gently guided into position by caring hands, and others where I have felt myself brace against touch that felt neither skilful nor caring. I have received some which offered me a sense of support and reassurance and others that took me beyond where I could comfortably breathe or felt able to say 'no'.

Similarly, I know students who love receiving hands-on assists and others whose life experiences make them feel anxious or triggered even in anticipating them. It can be worth remembering that students are not simply bodies to be placed in position but human beings with varying life experiences; that to support them in feeling safe we must offer them agency to choose if, how and when they receive touch.

My use of hands-on assists has changed over the years. More recently, I offer verbal cues as much as possible and ask permission if I feel that touch would offer useful guidance. Some teachers use permission cards enabling students to state clearly whether they want to be touched, which I think can be valuable.

If we are offering touch, we can be sensitive to the fact that before we connect with students physically, we are entering their energetic space surrounding them. Moving into this slowly and mindfully is important. If someone's eyes are closed, we can announce our presence calmly but audibly so that they have time to acknowledge it. If we are to offer them physical assistance, we ask for their permission before proceeding, where possible informing them of what we intend to do with them, for example, 'May I lift your hand?' or 'May I touch you here?'.

When touching another person, we can be sensitive to the fact that we are not just connecting with muscle and bone but with a fellow human being whose body will carry the imprints of their lived experience. The quality of our touch can respect and reflect this, guiding rather than moving with force, meeting the other with confidence, care and compassion rather than veering into what could be perceived as sensual or sexual.

When offering a modification, whether verbally or through touch, we can offer it as a suggestion so that students have agency to choose whether it is supportive or not. I often open with, 'May I offer you a suggestion?' as we explore a way of approaching a pose slightly differently, but then offer, 'Feel free to go back to where you were if that felt better'.

My concern with stronger physical assists that move students deeper into poses is that they suggest that bigger is better, that rather than working respectfully within our abilities and limitations we should strive to push beyond them. While I doubt any teacher sets out with the intention to harm their students through such assists, I've heard of numerous injuries, sometimes life-changing ones, from receiving them. This is not compassion in action.

REFLECTIONS

If you offer hands-on assists in your teaching:

- Do they support students in finding greater ease and tailor the practice to their needs?

- Do they guide them more deeply into a pose?

Presenting props

Props are a valuable tool in practising mindfully and compassionately. Whether using industry-made yoga props or reaching for a cushion, a thick book or a blanket, props offer the opportunity to find qualities of steadiness and ease that are central to our practice. At times, they offer a reference to where we are in space, sensing into our edges as we notice where our body meets a bolster or feel a blanket against our skin. At other times, they enable us to adapt a pose to our unique needs; like Goldilocks in the tale of the three bears, they offer the chance to find our sweet spot that feels 'just right' rather than 'too little' or 'too much'. This is self-care in action.

I know of many teachers (including myself) whose use of props has increased over their years of practising. Many students, however, have misconceptions about props which leave them either reluctant to use them or judgemental about doing so. I've seen students striving uncomfortably to achieve a perceived 'ideal' version of a pose and faces strained while hands reach for feet. There can be a notion that 'props = beginner, no props = advanced'.

In my beginners' yoga workshops, I ask participants how they feel when a teacher suggests they use a prop. Common responses are that they are 'rubbish', 'doing it wrong' even 'humiliated'. The consensus is that the teacher is saying that they are incapable of doing the 'real' pose and, therefore, 'bad' at yoga. They expressed feeling embarrassed and even ashamed for needing them when others don't.

How can we present props in a way that encourages people to care for themselves, to maximize the benefits of their practice without it feeling like we've told them to don stabilisers while everyone else is setting off to cycle the Tour de France?

SUGGESTIONS FOR PRESENTING PROPS

- *Personal experience*: Sharing how we as teachers benefit from using props in our own practice can highlight that their use and benefits are not restricted to beginners.

- *Props for all*: Incorporating practices where everyone uses props (e.g., a blanket under the torso to gently open the chest or a bolster supporting the torso in Child's Pose) can help reframe props as tools that support everyone.

- *Positively framing:* Framing choices from a place of positivity over deficiency. For example, consider the impact of hearing, 'If you enjoyed/benefited from the support of a block' rather than, 'If you needed the support of the block'. Similarly, suggesting, 'Don't be afraid to reach for a prop here' can subtly suggest that doing so is an act of courage, rather than a sign of inadequacy.

- *Relationship to support:* Props can offer valuable insights into our relationship to support, our ability to recognize when we need it and our willingness to access or ask for it. Self-sufficiency is celebrated in some cultures (as if strength is demonstrated through not needing external support), and I often wonder if this feeds into people's resistance. Offering points of inquiry can be interesting, particularly in longer held restorative poses, inviting students to notice how it feels to lean into support. Does it feel strange or familiar? Is there relief or resistance? Is it something they offer themselves permission for in life? Doing so can offer students valuable insights.

REFLECTION

- What is your own relationship with props and how do you incorporate and present them within your teaching?

Chapter 20

MOVING INTO STILLNESS

How and where we sequence *Śavāsana* and meditation can, of course, vary. As we saw earlier, a moment of mindful awareness at the start of our practice offers a way of landing and tuning into ourselves. At times, we might open a practice with a seated meditation or take it as a stand-alone practice. I'm a big fan of taking *Śavāsana* on its own in my personal practice, soaking up rest when it is needed. For many, it feels supportive to offer a meditation after *prāṇāyāma* and *Śavāsana*, enabling minds to feel more alert having soaked up conscious rest prior to it.

Śavāsana

I remember my niece, then aged about seven, informing me with delight about her yoga class at school. 'The best bit, Aunty Anna', she said, 'is that at the end you get to go to sleep!!!'. Despite common tendencies, the intention of *Śavāsana* is to remain calmly awake and aware. In our sleep-deprived culture, allowing students to soak up sleep can be compassion in action, but it can be helpful to highlight that this is not our intention.

In many ways *Śavāsana* is an open-awareness meditation, in which we tune into the nature of our experience without trying to shape it. For many, the body is more at ease lying down, but it could equally be taken as a seated meditation for those who prefer it.

While *Śavāsana* may initially appear to be an 'easy' pose, in which we do 'nothing', it is traditionally recognized as one of the most challenging. For many of us, standing on one leg is far easier than our minds staying present while lying in stillness without either sleepiness or distraction. As with many things, conscious rest requires regular practice and adequate preparation.

Śavāsana can be a welcome relief to some, but unfamiliar or challenging for others. In cultures where 'doing' and 'achieving' are markers of value, it is understandable that some either feel resistant to or avoid *Śavāsana,* feeling that being inactive holds no value. Educating students that 'doing nothing is actually doing something'[1] can be life-changing. We might remind students that this state of rest stimulates the parasympathetic nervous system, creating the conditions for healing and wellbeing, reducing our fear-based tendencies of thinking and accessing our intuitive wisdom. I had a yoga therapy client who was so averse to the concept of 'doing nothing' that we reframed it as 'active rest', offering him language that gave him permission to receive it.

The guidance we offer *in Śavāsana* supports students in understanding its purpose as well as navigating its challenges. It requires striking a balance between offering sufficient guidance and allowing space for silence. The length of time we allocate to *Śavāsana* can help students recognize its value rather than it seeming a box to be quickly ticked at the end of the 'real' practice.

Śavāsana offers a wonderful opportunity for practicing self-care. As teachers we can emphasize the importance of reaching for whatever allows comfort and ease, whether it be a bolster under the knees, the soft support of a blanket under the head or the warmth of one on top.

Traditionally, *Śavāsana* is taken lying on our backs, legs extended, feet wider than hips and arms resting by our side.

While this is comfortable for many, it isn't for all. Offering permission to take alternative positions (e.g., lying on our side or our belly, placing the legs on a chair) enables students to find the position that enables their body to access ease. For those who find lying supine vulnerable or anxiety inducing, being seated may be preferable; similarly, closing eyes is optional.

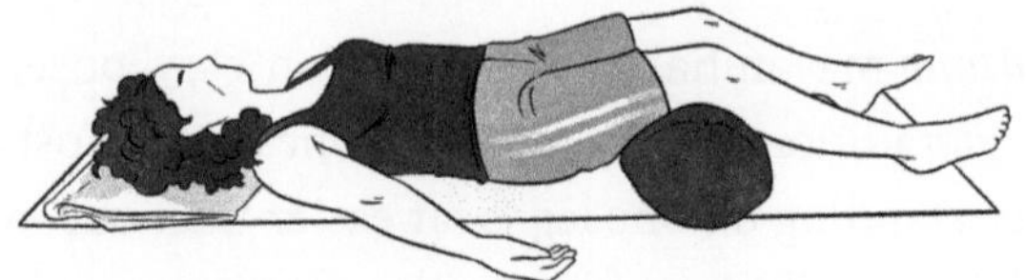

Traditional *Śavāsana*

Variations of Śavāsana

Side Lying *Śavāsana*

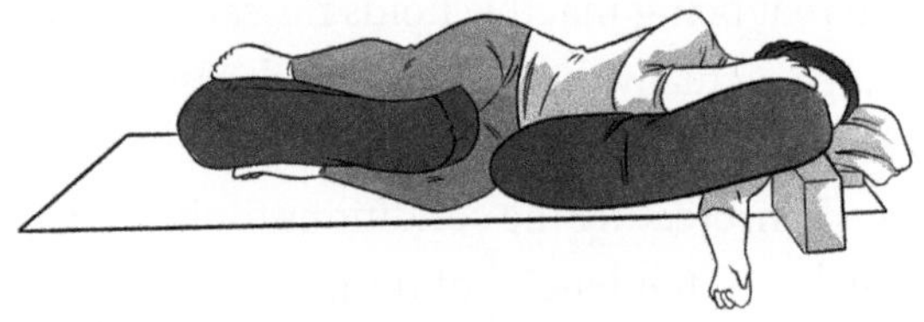

Side Lying *Śavāsana*

Place the head on sufficient support that the neck is aligned with the spine (here, this is created with a folded blanket over a flat block). Place some support between the knees (here, it is a bolster, but it could be folded blankets). Place a bolster between the belly and a brick in front of the face for the top arm to rest on.

Front Lying *Śavāsana*

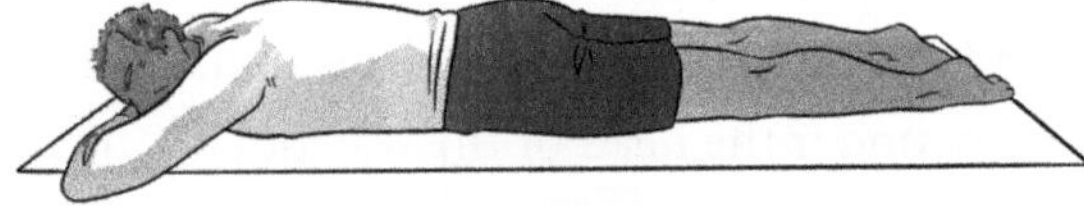

Front Lying *Śavāsana*

This can be as simple as lying on the belly, the hands making a support for the head as it turns to the side (turning the head at a half-way point). Alternatively, you could place two bolsters in a 'T' shape with the pelvis on the horizontal bolster and the torso over the vertical bolster, the head turned to the side. A rolled up blanket under the ankles in this version can offer greater comfort.

Legs on a chair

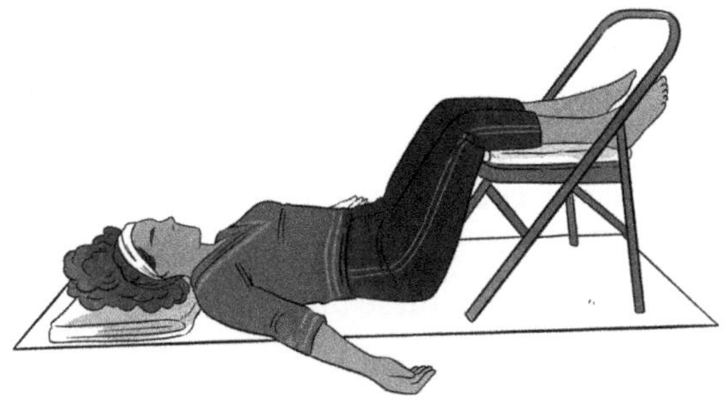

Legs on a Chair

Placing the legs over a chair (or a sofa or bed) can feel comfortable for many. Make sure that the back of the knees are supported by the chair. If the chair is quite hard, place a blanket over the chair for comfort. You may also roll up the blanket under the ankles. Placing the weight of a bolster over the shins can feel grounding for some.

Qualities that are beneficial in supporting rest are:

- sufficient support to offer comfort (it can be helpful to remind students that we are not seeking an active stretch here)

- warmth (covering with a blanket can be helpful)

- quietness (offering some time without instructions)

- darkness (for many, turning the lights low can be more comfortable than complete darkness, or using an eye pillow can be supportive)

- for many, weight feels helpful in feeling contained (e.g., the weight and warmth of being covered with a blanket, or the use of an eye pillow and sandbags, where appropriate).

While *Śavāsana* offers space for 'non-doing' it requires a careful balance between effort and ease. While the body is invited to let go of its holding, the mind is asked to remain open and present (rather than veering into the activity of thinking or the dullness of sleep).

As its name implies, *Śavāsana* (meaning 'Corpse Pose') is a practice of letting go. It offers preparation for our ultimate letting go, letting go of this body, this life, this last breath from a place of peaceful surrender. In the stillness of *Śavāsana* we practise letting go of our habitual doing, our tendencies towards achieving, fixing, changing and controlling. We practise opening to the life moving through us without trying to manipulate it.

Students' resistance to letting go is sometimes palpable. Some remain eager to seek active stretches, while others struggle to let go of a strong *ujjāyi* breath. Emphasizing this intention and what we might need to soften can bring awareness to these unconscious ways in which we seek to maintain 'control' and 'doing'.

Initially, it may be helpful to offer some guidance on where to place attention, perhaps starting with that which is most palpable (their connection to the earth and props that support them) and drawing towards the more subtle (e.g., sensations of letting go in the body and breath).

We sometimes think of *Śavāsana* as guiding students into a state of relaxation; however, as mindfulness and compassion became more integral to my teaching, instructions to 'relax' began to feel less helpful. As lovely as relaxation can sound, it can become another task to be achieved. 'Relaxation' might seem like a destination, a marker to judge ourselves against, whereas 'softening' or 'letting go' feels more a direction of travel to be explored.

We might sense a difference in tone between an instruction to 'relax your arm' and the more invitational language of noticing tension and 'exploring what *might* soften, even the slightest bit', or 'offering the body permission to soften, as much as it is willing or ready to' or 'softening the edges of what is holding'. Such language highlights that it is an exploration of possibilities rather than a demanding of outcomes. It offers an appreciation that moving towards a more relaxed state is not something to be rushed or demanded.

Here, we encourage softening, not only of the body and breath, but also of expectations and judgements that can arise when this is difficult. Sometimes, patterns of holding form a protection and we will find greater ease by meeting this with acceptance than feeling we are failing.

In the stillness, with less concrete factors to engage our attention, our minds can easily veer into thinking (I think I spent the first seven years of my practice thinking about what I would eat for dinner in *Śavāsana*!). As teachers, we can acknowledge that thoughts will arise but offer suggestions for meeting them, learning to be patient with our mind's need to keep 'doing'. We might even have a gentle word with them, suggesting 'dear mind, I appreciate your help, but in this moment, let us be right here and now'. We can invite students to sense the possibility of allowing their mind to rest back in a more spacious, kind awareness, one that *holds* their experience and allows them to gently observe what moves *through* it – sounds that arise and pass, sensations that come and go, the breath that flows, thoughts and feelings – without needing to leap onto, shape or react to it. It can feel a relief to many to sense that, just in this moment, they don't need to fix or change anything, they can just *be with* what is, and sensing that this is enough.

We can then, and most importantly, allow sufficient space and quietness for students to *be* with their experience without interruption or instruction.

Meditation

I'm often asked about the difference between mindfulness and meditation. Mindfulness is a type of meditation; however, not all meditation techniques are considered 'mindful' nor need to be seated.

Mindfulness can be thought of as an 'inclusive' form of meditation in that we include whatever moves through our awareness. Initially, we may choose a main focal point to anchor our attention (e.g., sounds, bodily sensations or breath); at other times, we can simply be open to whatever moves through our awareness (e.g., sounds, sensations, thoughts and feelings), sometimes known as 'open-awareness' meditation. We can practice mindfulness when sitting, lying down, walking and moving or in any activity in which we bring our full attention to our experience.

Some other meditation techniques can be thought of as 'exclusive' in that awareness is directed solely towards one focal point (e.g., a mantra, an object or visualization) with the intention of excluding other stimulus and, therefore, focusing the mind.

While mindfulness invites us to open to our experience *as it is*, other techniques often seek to shape our experience in a particular direction (e.g., stimulating relaxation, balancing *cakras*, cultivating loving kindness). Both inclusive and exclusive meditation techniques hold value, and

I offer both in my teaching; however, it can be helpful to understand their differences.

For many students the word 'meditation' can conjure up images of sitting in lotus position for lengthy periods, the mind blissfully peaceful or void of thoughts. Such myths can make meditation feel daunting and inaccessible, as well as leave students feeling that they are failing when their busy mind continues to 'interrupt' their practice.

Dispelling such myths is helpful; indeed we don't even need to name a practice as meditation, we can simply invite students to tune into a particular anchor over a period that feels manageable.

As always, we want to meet our students where they are. There is little to be gained in suggesting that someone new to meditation sit cross-legged for 30 minutes. Offering just a few minutes (2–5 minutes) of meditation can be impactful, building the length progressively, as appropriate.

Supporting students in finding comfort makes all the difference in their ability to access meditation for extended periods. While exploring unpleasant sensations can form a part of our practice, we wish to reduce unnecessary elements of it. Our intention is for our body to offer a steady foundation, rather than constantly shifting due to discomfort, and our mind to be able to rest on our focal point rather than being dominated by feelings of pain.

Offering either a mindful, or compassionate Body Scan can be a lovely way of offering students an extended meditation while lying down, a position that for many feels more comfortable than sitting for a longer period.

Sitting upright in meditation holds many benefits, enabling the body to reflect the qualities of heart/mind that we seek to cultivate (e.g., alert, wakeful, open yet relaxed) and reduces tendencies towards falling asleep, which can happen when we are lying down (although I can testify it's still possible to fall asleep in a seated meditation when tired!). However, if we or our students are unable to sit due to health reasons, practices can be taken in any position that allows for comfort.

Images of meditators sitting cross-legged can leave some students believing that this is the 'ideal' or 'real' meditation posture, resulting in them striving to attain it despite the discomfort they experience. Offering students a range of options and presenting them with equal validity can make seated meditation more accessible.

We might highlight that we are looking for certain qualities in our posture and that these can be accessed in a range of positions. Key elements that we are seeking in our seated posture are for our:

- lower body to feel steady and grounded

- spine to feel upright

- chest to feel open rather than collapsed

- hands to rest in such a way that our shoulders can relax (using a blanket on the lap can support this)

- chin to very slightly drop so that the back of the neck is long.

For many, sitting with hips higher than knees and feet is supportive. If sitting for prolonged periods, placing a cushion on the lap to rest the hands or tucking the hands into a blanket around the waist can allow the shoulders to feel more supported and relaxed. When we are still, there can be a tendency for body temperature to drop so wrapping a blanket either around the lower or full body can be helpful.

Common seated meditation postures are outlined below.

Sitting on a chair

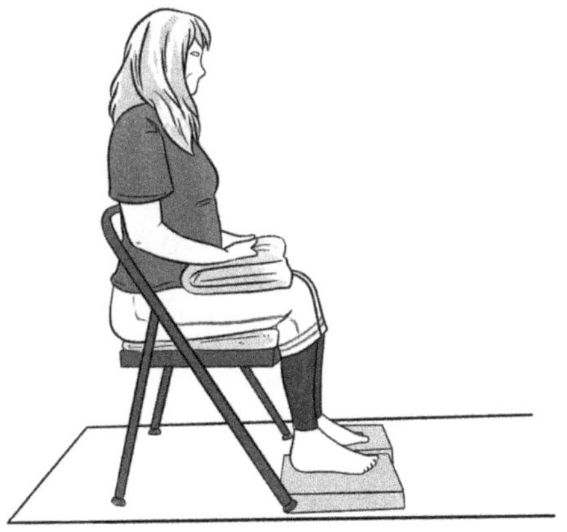

Meditation Sitting on a Chair

- Place both feet on the ground or on blocks or cushions if this feels more grounding.

- Sit a little away from the back of your chair so that you have the natural curves in your spine. If this is challenging to sustain, you might place some cushions behind your back for support.

- Hands can be placed on your legs or on a folded blanket or cushion on your legs if this helps the shoulders feel more relaxed.

Kneeling

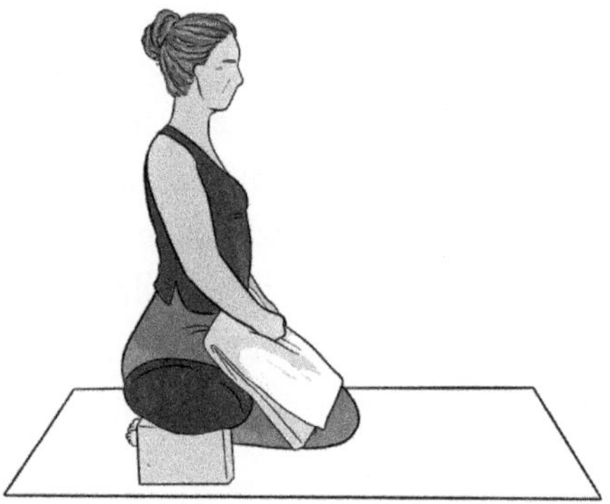

Meditation Kneeling

- Place as many cushions or yoga blocks as you need underneath your seat to gain sufficient height and comfort. Sit astride the support with your shins on the floor and the support under your sit bones. Alternatively, as illustrated here, create a structure (here, a bolster supported by two bricks) to create a meditation 'bench', placing the feet behind you.

- If this places strain on your ankles, place a rolled-up towel/blanket under your ankles to reduce the intensity of stretch.

- Hands can rest on thighs or on a folded blanket in your lap.

Sukhāsana

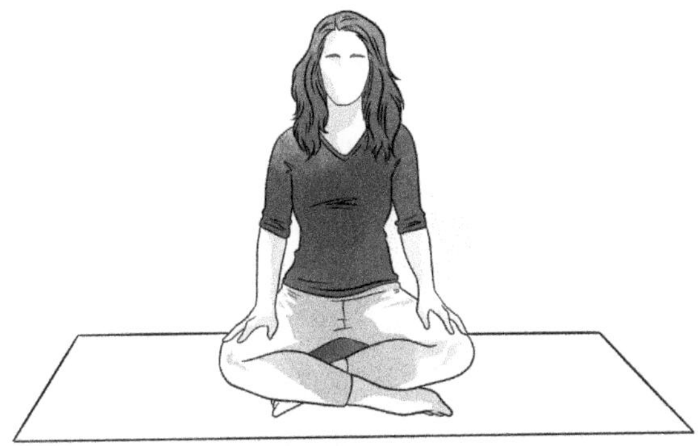

Meditation *Sukhāsana*

- Place sufficient support under your seat (e.g., cushions or blocks) so that your hips are higher than your knees.

- Ideally, have your knees on the ground or supported by cushions.

- Sit towards the front edge of the cushion so that the pelvis tilts slightly forward and the spine lengthens (offering your lower back space rather than rounding).

- Hands can rest on thighs, a folded blanket in your lap or tucked into a blanket around your waist.

Siddhāsana

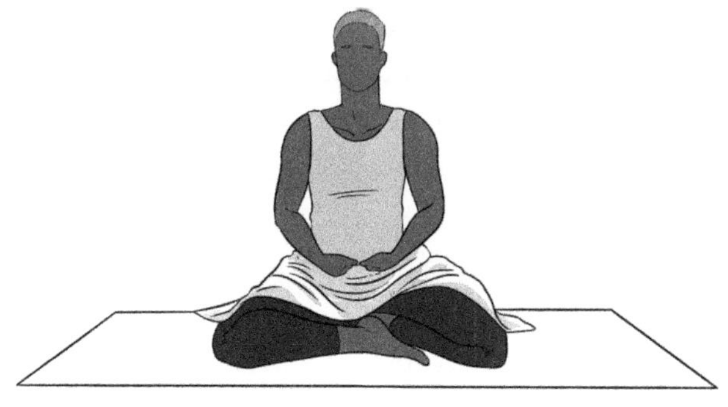

Meditation *Siddhāsana*

- As with *Sukhāsana* it can be helpful to have sufficient support under the seat so that the hips are higher than the knees.

- Bend one knee so that the heal of that foot comes near to the groin.

- Bend the other knee so that foot comes close to the other foot.

- Sit towards the front edge of the cushion so that the pelvis tilts slightly forward and the spine lengthens (offering your lower back space rather than rounding).

- Hands can rest on thighs or a folded blanket in your lap or be tucked into a blanket around your waist.

With both cross-legged variations, it can be beneficial to change the cross of the legs in different sittings, to avoid always having the same shin in front to allow for greater balance.

Mindful meditations

The Body Scan

When so many of us move through life lost in thought, the Body Scan offers space to reconnect with the body. We might offer a short version at the start of a practice to help 'land' in the body. At other times, we might offer it for an extended period, either as a stand-alone practice, or at the end in *Śavāsana*.

Here, we scan attention through the body in a systematic order (e.g., toes to head or head to toes), tuning into the sensations experienced at each stage. When teaching, it can be helpful to highlight that the Body Scan isn't intended as a relaxation technique (nor is relaxation a preferred outcome), but rather as an opportunity to bring the attitudes of mindful awareness to our experience of the body, meeting it is at is, with curiosity, care, patience and acceptance. In my experience, sometimes I meet areas of tension that soften slightly as soon as they are seen, while others feel the impact of being met with acceptance and compassion as they remain.

Below is an outline of an extended Body Scan (that could take between 20–30 minutes).

- Find a comfortable position lying down on your back in *Śavāsana* or in an alternative posture if more comfortable. Suggested support would be a pillow or a bolster under the knees, a thin cushion or blanket under the head, and a blanket to cover for warmth.

- Sense the body as a whole, its connection to the earth and the space around you. If anything needs to shift to be slightly more comfortable allow for this.

- Rest your awareness on your breath for a moment without trying to shape it; simply observe its natural ebb and flow wherever you sense it most easily (e.g., the belly, chest, throat or nose).

- Now, systematically guide awareness through the body, spending a few moments with each body part. Tune into the sensations you experience there (e.g., coolness, heat, pressure, space, contact of clothing or props, tension, ease, tingling, numbness or simply lack of sensation).

- Notice how you are meeting the body (e.g., judgements, expectations or striving for a particular outcome) and see where you can bring in attitudes of mindful awareness.

- When you notice the mind has wandered (as it tends to do frequently), guide it back to the body. There's no need to judge yourself for this, inherent in the practice is noticing when we have wandered into thinking and gently, patiently returning to presence.

- At times we will also notice mental and emotional states. We might feel bored, sleepy, agitated or peaceful. See if you can observe these in the same way as you do the physical sensations, with care and interest. You might be curious about where you feel an emotion in the body (e.g., does agitation make you fidgety, or anger express itself in the chest or belly?).

- Urges might arise (e.g., to scratch an itch, to move, to finish the practice early). See if you can observe these urges without acting on them. Of course, if, after a while, you realize it's wise and compassionate to move (rather than the desire coming from the mind, unconsciously eager for something to 'do'), you might do so, but perhaps the urge passes.

- Once you have scanned through each body part, broaden your focus again to observe the body as a whole, observing the shifting, changing nature of sensations and aliveness moving through you.

- Afterwards, take a moment to reflect on what you noticed physically, mentally and emotionally during the practice.

Depending on the time available and a student's capacity for awareness, we might, at times, focus on larger areas of the body (e.g., tuning into the whole foot, then the lower leg or even both hands at the same time) or smaller areas (e.g., sensing into one toe at a time before the sole of the foot, the top of the foot, the heel).

In journeying through our inner landscape, we sense how 'our body' isn't one constant entity, but rather a multitude of varying experiences; some feel pleasant to inhabit, some we habitually zone out from, others may be dominated by tension or pain. We gain insights into our relationship with our body, whether befriending, ignoring or battling with it. It took me years of practice to realize that, while I could often remain interested and engaged through much of the practice, my attention would forever wander when my attention drew to my abdomen, regardless of the direction my attention travelled!

While the intention of the Body Scan is to stay awake and aware, many of us are deprived of adequate rest and it's common to fall asleep. Exploring the practice with the eyes open, seated or even standing can be helpful alternatives. That said, we can also be compassionate to ourselves and students if we do fall asleep, allowing for this act of self-care, if it is needed.

The Compassionate Body Scan

The Compassionate Body Scan follows a similar format to the Body Scan (i.e., systematically scanning through and meeting each body part and opening to how it feels), but then adds a layer of action by offering kindness towards each part. There are different ways that we can express care and kindness towards the body, we might offer it soothing touch or caring words of understanding and appreciation (e.g., 'Dear mouth, thank you for all you've allowed me to say and taste today', or, 'Dear hands, I know you've done a lot of typing today').

Personally, I love a version shared by Sharon Salzberg in *Real Love*,[2] in which she invites us to meet and open to each body part, noticing how it feels, before wishing it peace and happiness (e.g., 'May my head be happy. May it feel peaceful'). Once we have taken our attention throughout the whole body, I like to sense the whole again (i.e., body, mind and heart) offering silently, 'May *I* be happy, may *I* feel peaceful'.

I find the Compassionate Body Scan a particularly helpful practice when people are unwell or experiencing difficulty within their body or when offering kindness to themselves as a whole feels challenging. For some, offering kindness to individual body parts (e.g., wishing the feet ease) feels an easier place to start than to themselves as a whole.

Another lovely practice to cultivate feelings of connection and gratitude for the body can be to scan the body and simply offer 'thank you' towards each body part.

Mindfulness of Breathing

As the name implies, Mindfulness of Breathing uses the breath as the anchor for awareness. Here, we're not seeking to shape the breath in any way (e.g., slowing or deepening it), but rather observing its natural flow as we find it. Personally, I often find that simply in becoming aware of my breathing it changes slightly, but it is more a case of it finding its comfortable form and rhythm than something I am consciously doing. Rather than *thinking* about the breath, we are tuning into our sensory experience of it. We might think of resting a light attention on the breath rather than scrutinizing it intently. We are still open to the fullness of our experience (e.g., aware of sounds, sensations, thoughts and feelings), but the breath is in the foreground.

At times, we might take mindful breathing for a few breaths to centre and gather. At others, we could take it for an extended practice over 10–30 minutes. A longer practice is generally taken seated (finding a comfortable posture that supports easeful breathing), but, if this is not accessible, it could be taken lying down. As with any meditation, the eyes could be either closed or a soft gaze cast low.

Within some Buddhist traditions, Mindfulness of Breathing is taken in four stages. If we were sitting for 20 minutes, we could set a timer to mark each five-minute stage as follows:

1. Softly, silently counting after each exhale, aware of the space that follows the exhale (e.g., inhale, exhale '1', inhale, exhale '2'). The counting can be helpful for many in both maintaining focus and noticing when it has veered. If we lose count (because the mind has wandered) or we count to 10 (which can be surprisingly more challenging than we think), we simply restart at 1.

2. As per above but placing the count before each inhale, anticipating the breath flowing in (e.g., '1' inhale, exhale, '2' inhale, exhale).

3. Dropping the count and simply observing the natural flow of the breath in and out.

4. Focusing attention at the nostrils, tuning into the sensations as the breath enters and leaves the body.

An alternative way to take the practice is to allow attention to rest on different elements of the breath, sometimes broadening and sometimes narrowing the focal point of our awareness. Again, I would suggest offering sufficient time at each stage so that there is a clear focal point for a few minutes at a time, rather than feeling attention darting around. Some suggestions are to direct awareness towards:

- wherever the breath is sensed most easily (this will differ from person to person; common places are the abdomen, chest, throat and nose)

- specific locations within the body (e.g., sensing the breath at the abdomen)

- the tone and texture of the breath (e.g., its speed, depth, texture, temperature)

- sensations of expansion and contraction as the breath moves through the body

- elements of the breath (e.g., the inhalation, the exhalation, the turning points between the breath flowing in and out)

- exploring the whole journey of the breath from start to end

- the felt sense of the whole body breathing.

The beauty of using the breath as an anchor is that, like the body, it is always with us. In moments when we feel thrown off centre, we can easily access it to return to presence.

Compassionate Breathing

With the Compassionate Breathing practice, we imagine imbuing the breath with a quality of kindness. Here, we might imagine the breath like a dear friend that we can be soothed by. Again, this is a practice that we would ideally take sitting so the chest area is more open, but it could be taken lying down (or in any moment in life when it feels supportive).

- Take a moment to find a comfortable posture that supports easeful breathing. Choose whether you would like to close your eyes or rest your gaze low.

- Bring your attention to the chest and sense qualities of warmth and care here. If helpful, you could place one or both hands on the chest to have a visceral sense of these qualities as well as a more perceptible sense of the breath under the palms.

- Connect with the flow of the breath and allow it to become smooth and steady. You might imagine it like a soft, soothing wave that gently massages you from the inside.

- Imagine with each inhale the heart centre is filled with loving kindness. With each exhale its kindness radiates within you, the body softening to receive it with ease.

At times, we might guide the breath towards a place that is holding or hurting; at others, to the whole body. There may be times when the heart's kindness is directed inwardly towards ourselves and others where we use the exhale to imagine extending kindness externally to others or the world at large.

Loving Kindness Meditation (Metta Bhavana)

While there are many variations of this practice, the intention is the same, cultivating feelings of loving kindness and directing them both inwardly towards ourselves, and outwardly towards others. Traditionally it is taken in five stages, offering kindness to:

1. Ourselves.

2. Someone we find it easy and uncomplicated to offer kindness towards (e.g., a friend, loved one, a mentor, even a pet).

3. A neutral person (e.g., someone we don't have strong feelings of like or dislike toward, perhaps someone we see regularly on a journey, someone working in our local shop, or a bus driver).

4. A difficult person (e.g., someone whose behaviour causes us difficulty). When choosing a difficult person, avoid choosing someone who could feel traumatic or triggering to connect with. Instead, think of someone who feels manageable, that we feel annoyed or disgruntled by rather than someone who could feel overwhelming to sit with.

5. All four together (e.g., ourselves, the friend or mentor, the neutral and difficult person) before incrementally broadening our circle of caring to encompass all beings (e.g., imagining those in our street, town, country, continent, the whole world).

This can be a powerful practice for cultivating a sense of our common humanity. Particularly with the neutral and difficult people, it can remind us that everyone has layers of complexity that we don't see on the surface; that we all have our hopes and dreams, our triggers and difficulties. It doesn't ask us to agree with or condone someone's behaviour, but to appreciate that people are complex beings whose behaviours are influenced by their histories and conditioning; that they, like us, are often steered by a desire to be safe and happy, even if we don't agree with their way of going about it.

There are numerous ways that we might offer loving kindness. Often, within this practice, it is undertaken through the repetition of phrases of loving kindness. Potential phrases could include 'May I/you/we…'

- be well

- be safe

- be happy

- be healthy

- be peaceful

- be kind to myself/yourself/ourselves

- lovingly accept myself/yourself/ourselves as I am/you are/we are

- live with ease and kindness

- be filled with loving kindness.

If sharing in a group setting, we might choose three or four phrases that feel most appropriate. If taking for ourselves or working one-to-one, we might explore which words resonate most. By selecting phrases that we connect with personally, we are more likely to remain connected to the intention of the practice rather than the words becoming mechanical in their repetition.

In recent months, the phrases that I like to offer are:

- May I be well in body, heart and mind.

- May I know peace and contentment.

- May I be open to and grateful for what's good in my life.

- May I meet life's difficulties with compassion.

When life is challenging, either for ourselves or others, adding the words, 'in the midst of this', may feel helpful in cultivating a quality of equanimity.

Alternative ways that we could imagining sending kindness could include:

- Imagining our heart filling with loving kindness as we inhale and directing it towards ourselves or the other/s as we exhale. People who are visual may like to connect with a colour that they associate with kindness and imagine directing this inwardly and outwardly.

- Wishing each person something practical that would make their day and hearts more easeful such as wishing the bus driver, 'May you have friendly passengers today', or the post person, 'May you have comfortable shoes'. This version often makes me smile.

The number of stages we include and length of time allocated to each can vary. At times, we might rest our attention only on ourselves. If sharing with someone new to the practice, we might include the first three people and build up to the difficult one when more experienced. In a class setting, we might offer it towards the shared group, sensing our place in the collective group practising. While it is traditionally a seated practice, we could easily take it while walking or offering kindness to those sitting in the train carriage with us.

It's interesting that within the Buddhist tradition, starting with ourselves was considered the easiest, least complicated option; however, for many, this feels the most challenging. Given this, some people may find it helpful to begin with someone their heart opens easily to *before* offering kindness towards themselves. On days when we struggle to offer kindness to ourselves, we might imagine someone who cares for and sees the good in us (even a pet) directing loving kindness towards us.

It can be interesting to reflect on which stage we find our attention is most or least focused, which elements our hearts easily connect to and which feel challenging. Perhaps when meeting the difficult one, we need reminding to also have self-compassion, if it understandably feels challenging. Again, we practise bringing the qualities of mindful awareness (e.g., patience, acceptance, non-judgement) towards ourselves in the practice.

Transitioning towards daily life

The end of any practice offers a valuable opportunity to pause before reengaging with our everyday lives. As with all transitionary periods, it can be helpful to linger here a little, to respect its potency.

Just as we offer students time to land and arrive at the start of their practice, we can offer time here to notice the residue their practice has left; time to tune into how they *now* feel in body, heart, mind. What messages do these different layers offer? Do they feel more integrated than at the start?

We might invite students to notice anything they feel they would like to carry with them as they step off the mat. Whether it be a little more ease, steadiness, strength or peace, inviting them to pause with it for a short moment, offering it time to be seen and felt, to notice how and where it plays out within the body, heart, mind and to acknowledge their capacity to cultivate this for themselves.

We might drop in points of inquiry while minds are quieter, hearts more open and we have greater capacity to listen to intuitive insights that often arise when nervous systems are calmer. This might be an invitation to consider:

- how the theme of the practice could be woven into their life off the mat

- a small way in which they might offer themselves some kindness or sense of balance that day

- a person or place that offers them a sense of steadiness and taking a moment to feel grateful for this

- any insights that arose in the quietness

- anything that needs acknowledging, nourishing or tending to as they return to their daily lives.

Doing so can reinforce that the benefits of our practice are meant to be felt as much *off* the mat as on it.

If teaching in a group setting, even the act of putting props away can be framed as an opportunity to practise loving kindness, playing a part in leaving the space feeling peaceful and supportive for those who will practice after us.

CLOSING THOUGHTS AND HOPES

In our technological age of fast speed, heightened stimulation and instant results, it is easy to see how people's yoga practice can follow suit. It can feel a rare and precious gift to be offered space and permission to slow, still and quieten; to let our precious attention fold back inwards towards ourselves.

Our worth is so often gauged by how much we have done and what we have achieved that many of us are doing too much; we literally rest less and are *restless*, exhausted but struggling to sleep. When more value is placed on our output than our input, our yoga practice can become yet another thing to be 'done' rather than offering ourselves space to 'be', to care for, to nourish and receive. We all need spaces where we do and talk less and learn to listen more deeply.

Social media platforms frequently present images of unattainable perfection and fuel feelings of comparisons and competition, creating a vicious cycle between striving and lacking. I recently had a student arrive in class with a tripod and camera asking if I minded her recording herself while she practised. While she was understanding and respectful of my reasons for not allowing this, I found her request concerning.

Our yoga practice is not a performance to be seen or broadcast, nor its success gauged by our physical prowess or the number of likes that it gets. We all need spaces where we can drop the masks we feel we need to present to the world; places where we can safely, sensitively open to our vulnerabilities, celebrate our uniqueness; where we can recognize our validity in belonging and our inherent interconnectedness.

Rather than bodies becoming entities that we drag around but are disconnected from or that we feel need to be shaped or battled with, our practice invites us to reconnect with and befriend them, to learn how to navigate their varied landscapes and listen to their deeply held wisdom. We need reminders to value, nurture and nourish them.

My hope is that, through our practice and teaching, there are more people who are awake, aware and connected to their hearts; who recognize what balance feels like and how to return to it when life throws them off centre; people who are sufficiently rested and resourced to bring wise, compassionate action into this world that so very much needs it.

Excerpt from the poem *The Fruits of Practice*

by Danna Faulds

… Practice isn't about achieving
a goal. It's not a means to pole-
vault over suffering. Practice
is my way of looking life in
the face and saying yes to all
its disparate gifts. Practice
keeps me awake when I would
sleep, and reminds me it's
the journey, unfolding in this
very moment, it's the journey
that reveals the truth, and
not the destination.

BIBLIOGRAPHY

Analayo, B. (2019) *Satipatthana, The Direct Path to Realization*. Cambridge: Windhorse Publications.

Boccio, F.J. (2004) *Mindfulness Yoga: An Awakened Union of Breath, Body, and Mind*. Somerville: Wisdom Publications.

Brach, T. (2003) *Radical Acceptance*. New York: Bantam Dell, A Division of Random House, Inc.

Brach, T. (2013) *True Refuge*. London: Hay House UK Ltd.

Burch, V. (2008) *Living Well with Pain and Illness*. London: Piatkus.

Desikachar, T.K.V. (2003) *Reflections on Yoga Sūtra-s of Patañjali*. Chennai: Krishnamacharya Yoga Mandiram.

Farhi, D. (2004) *Bringing Yoga To Life*. New York: HarperCollins.

Feldman, C. (2017) *Boundless Heart, The Buddha's Path of Kindness, Compassion, Joy, and Equanimity*. Boulder, CO: Shambhala Publications, Inc.

Forbes, B. (2011) *Yoga for Emotional Balance*. Boston, MA: Shambhala Publications, Inc.

Geller, S. (2013) 'Therapeutic Presence: An Essential Way of Being.' In Cooper, M., Schmid, P.F., O'Hara, M. & Bohart, A.C. (Eds) *The Handbook of Person-Centred Psychotherapy and Counselling*, 2nd edition. London: Palgrave Macmillan.

Germer, C. (2009) *The Mindful Path to Self-Compassion*. New York: The Guilford Press.

Gilbert., P & Choden (2015) *Mindful Compassion*, London: Constable & Robinson Ltd.

Gilbert, P. (2013) *The Compassionate Mind* London: Constable.

Gokhale, P. (2020) *The Yogasūtra of Patañjali*. Abingdon: Routledge.

Hanh, T.N. (2011) *Your True Home*. Boston, MA: Shambhala Publications, Inc.

Hanson, R. (2009) *Buddha's Brain*. Oakland, CA: New Harbinger Publications, Inc.

Kabat-Zinn, J. (2004) *Full Catastrophe Living*. London: Piatkus.

Kornfield, J. (2002) *A Path With Heart*. New York: Ebury Publishing.

Le Page, J. & Le Page, L. (2014) *Mudras for Healing and Transformation*. Fort Lauderdale: Fl. Integrative Yoga Therapy.

Moss, H. (2018) *The Practice of Mindful Yoga*. London: Leaping Hare Press.

Neff, K. (2011) *Self Compassion*. London: Hodder & Stoughton Ltd.

Neff, K. & Germer, C. (2018) *The Mindful Self-Compassion Workbook*. New York: The Guilford Press.

Porges, S. (2017) *The Pocket Guide to The Polyvagal Theory*. New York: W.W. Norton & Company, Inc.

Roy, R. & Charlton, D. (2019) *Embodying the Yoga Sutra*. London: YogaWords.

Salzberg, S (1995) *Loving Kindness*. Boston: Shambhala Publications, Inc.

Salzberg, S. (2017) *Real Love*. London: Bluebird.

Satchidananda (2008) *The Yoga Sutras of Patanjali*. Buckingham, VA: Integral Yoga Publications.

Siegel, D. (2017) *Mind: A Journey into the Heart of Being Human*. New York: W.W. Norton & Company.

Van Der Kolk, B. (2015) *The Body Keeps the Score*. London: Penguin.

Wall Kimmerer, R. (2013) *Braiding Sweetgrass*. London: Penguin.

Williams, M. & Penman, D. (2011) *Mindfulness: A Practical Guide to Finding Peace in a Frantic World*. London: Piatkus.

Williams, M. & Penman, D. (2023) *Deeper Mindfulness: Rediscover Calm in a Chaotic World*. London: Piatkus.

ENDNOTES

Introduction

1   Coleman Barks (Trans), 'A Mouse and a Frog' In *The Essential Rumi* (HarperCollins, 1995), p.80.
2   Tara Brach, PhD, *Radical Acceptance* (Bantam Books, 2003).

Section 1

1   See www.tsyp.yoga.
2   Ranju Roy and David Charlton, *Embodying the Yoga Sutra* (Pinter & Martin Ltd, 2019), p.28.

Chapter 1

1   Ranju Roy and David Charlton, *Embodying the Yoga Sutra* (Pinter & Martin Ltd, 2019).
2   Ranju Roy and David Charlton, *Embodying the Yoga Sutra* (Pinter & Martin Ltd, 2019), p.225.
3   Ranju Roy and David Charlton, *Embodying the Yoga Sutra* (Pinter & Martin Ltd, 2019), p.257.
4   Thich Nhat Hanh, *Your True Home* (Shambhala Publications, Inc, 2011), p.297.
5   See https://brenebrown.com/articles/2022/05/09/creating-space.
6   Jack Kornfield, *A Path With Heart* (Eury Publishing, 2002), p.107.
7   Jon Kabat-Zinn, *Full Catastrophe Living* (Piatkus, 2004), p.33.
8   See www.socratic-method.com/quote-meanings-interpretations/carl-rogers-the-curious-paradox-is-that-when-i-accept-myself-just-as-i-am-then-i-can-change#google_vignette?utm_content=cmp-true.
9   Jack Kornfield, *A Path with Heart* (Eury Publishing, 2002), p.36.
10   Rick Hanson, PhD, *Buddha's Brain* (New Harbinger Publications, Inc. 2009), p.68.
11   Daniel J. Siegel, MD, *Mind: a Journey into the Heart of Being Human* (W.W. Norton & Company, 2017), p.172.
12   Jon Kabat-Zinn, *Wherever You Go, There You Are.* (Piatkus Books, 2007), p.30.

Chapter 2

1   Tara Brach PH.D, *Radical Acceptance* (Bantam Books, 2003), p.27.
2   Paul Gilbert, *The Compassionate Mind* (Constable & Robinson Ltd, 2013), p.217.
3   Paul Gilbert & Choden, *Mindful Compassion* (Constable & Robinson Ltd, 2013), p.103.
4   Kristin Neff, PhD, *Self Compassion* (Hodder & Stoughton, 2011), p.42.
5   Paul Gilbert, *The Compassionate Mind* (Constable & Robinson Ltd, 2013), p.24.
6   Robin Wall Kimmerer, *Braiding Sweetgrass* (Penguin Books, 2013), p.94.

Section 2

1   Bessel Van Der Kolk, *The Body Keeps The Score* (Penguin Books, 2015), p.283.

Chapter 4

1   Jack Kornfield, *A Path With Heart* (Eury Publishing, 2002), p.10.

Chapter 6

1   Tara Brach, PhD, *Radical Acceptance* (Bantam Books, 2003), p.62.
2   See https://www.dhammatalks.org/suttas/AN/AN8_6.html.
3   Jon Kabat-Zinn, *Full Catastrophe Living* (Piatkus, 2004), pp.126–7.

Chapter 7

1   Sharon Salzberg, Real Love (Bluebird / Pan Macmillan, 2017), p.16.
2   Tara Brach, PhD, *True Refuge* (Hay House Publishers, 2013), p.118.
3   Paul Gilbert & Choden, *Mindful Compassion* (Constable & Robinson Ltd, 2013), p.362.
4   Kristin Neff, PhD and Christopher Germer, PhD, *The Mindful Self-Compassion Workbook* (The Guilford Press, 2018), pp.34–5.
5   Stephen W. Porges, *The Pocket Guide to The Polyvagal Theory* (W.W. Norton & Company, 2017).
6   Rick Hanson, PhD, *Buddha's Brain* (New Harbinger Publications, Inc. 2009), p.68.

Chapter 8

1   See https://centerforliving.org/boundaries-one-path-to-respectful-relationships-in-recovery-and-beyond.

Section 3

1   Donna Farhi, *Bringing Yoga To Life* (HarperCollins, 2003), p.193.

Chapter 11

1   Stephen W. Porges, *The Pocket Guide to The Polyvagal Theory* (W.W. Norton & Company, 2017).
2   Dr Shari Geller 'Therapeutic Presence: An Essential Way of Being.' In Cooper, M., Schmid, P.F., O'Hara, M. & Bohart, A.C. (Eds) *The Handbook of Person-Centred Psychotherapy and Counselling* (Palgrave Macmillan, 2013, 2nd ed.).
3   Dr Shari Geller 'Therapeutic Presence: An Essential Way of Being.' In Cooper, M., Schmid, P.F., O'Hara, M. & Bohart, A.C. (Eds) *The Handbook of Person-Centred Psychotherapy and Counselling* (Palgrave Macmillan, 2013, 2nd ed.).

Chapter 17

1   Tara Brach, PhD, *Radical Acceptance* (Bantam Books, 2003), p.91.
2   Kristin Neff, PhD and Christopher Germer, PhD, *The Mindful Self-Compassion Workbook* (The Guilford Press, 2018), p.33.
3   Jack Kornfield, *A Path With Heart* (Eury Publishing, 2002), p.12.
4   See www.healthline.com/health/hugging-benefits#7.-Hugs-help-you-communicate-with-others.

Chapter 18

1   Donna Farhi, *Bringing Yoga To Life* (HarperCollins, 2003), p.55.

Chapter 20

1   Thich Nhat Hanh, *Your True Home* (Shambhala Publications, Inc, 2011), p.297.
2   Sharon Salzbert, *Real Love* (Bluebird / Pan Macmillan, 2017), p.76.